Alzheimer's disease is a degenerative brain disease which has major social consequences for the individuals affected and for those who are emotionally and/or physically close to them. The role which language plays in such relationships stands at the center of this book. In contrast to traditional analyses carried out by psycholinguists, neurologists, and speech pathologists, with speech samples elicited in clinical settings, Heidi Ehernberger Hamilton examines language in the life of one elderly female Alzheimer's patient, from an interactional sociolinguistic perspective. The language of open-ended, naturally occurring conversations between the patient and the author, over four-and-one-half years, is investigated not only in an attempt to understand how the patient's communicative abilities and disabilities are related to each other and how they change over time, but, importantly, how they are influenced by both preemptive and reactive communicative behaviors on the part of the patient's healthy interlocutor. This "personal and particular" study of conversations with one Alzheimer's patient is offered as a humanistic approach to language loss. It is one in which communicative breakdowns are analyzed not separately from details about the patient, her conversational partners, and the setting, nor from relevant social facts which may influence interactions, that is, one in which language disability is seen as a human problem within multiple linguistic and social contexts.

Conversations with an Alzheimer's patient

Conversations with an Alzheimer's patient

An interactional sociolinguistic study

Heidi Ehernberger Hamilton

Department of Linguistics, Georgetown University

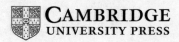

Published by the Press Syndicate of the University of Cambridge
The Pitt Building, Trumpington Street, Cambridge CB2 1RP
40 West 20th Street, New York, NY 10011-4211, USA
10 Stamford Road, Oakleigh, Melbourne 3166, Australia

First published 1994

Printed in Great Britain at the University Press, Cambridge

A catalogue record for this book is available from the British Library

Library of Congress cataloguing in publication data

Hamilton, Heidi Ehernberger.
Conversations with an Alzheimer's patient: an interactional
sociolinguistic study / Heidi Ehernberger Hamilton.
    p.   cm.
Includes bibliographical references (p.   ) and index.
ISBN 0 521 42101 2 (hardback)
1. Alzheimer's disease – Patients – Language – Case studies.
2. Language attrition – Case studies.   3. Sociolinguistics – Case
Studies.   I. Title.
RC523.H35   1994
618.97′6831 – dc20   93–1373   CIP

ISBN 0 521 42101 2 hardback

UP

for Dan
who challenges me to balance
intellect with creativity and care

Contents

Acknowledgments

It would be impossible to mention all of the people who either directly or indirectly have contributed to this book and the Ph.D. dissertation which forms the basis of it. My sincere thanks go to each and every one of them, although only a few can be named here.

I am truly grateful for those responsible for awarding me a Georgetown University Fellowship which enabled me to study within the intellectually stimulating and collegial environment of the Georgetown Department of Linguistics. There I came to know and respect some very talented professors and students.

I am indebted to Dr. Deborah Tannen, my dissertation adviser and mentor in every conceivable sense of the word, for sharing her humanistic vision of linguistics with me. Deborah's continuing expression of confidence in my abilities over the years has been of critical importance. Other early and lasting influences came from Dr. Deborah Schiffrin, Dr. Roger Shuy, and Dr. Ralph Fasold who, by example, taught me a great deal about how to combine high levels of scholarship with a sense of purpose and responsibility toward the solution of real-world problems. Fellow students whose discussions I will always cherish include Liz Lanza, Susan Hoyle, and Branca Ribeiro.

I am also grateful to Nikolas Coupland, Justine Coupland, and Howard Giles, for their early interest in my work on language and Alzheimer's disease. Their conviction that there was potential in my very early drafts and analyses encouraged me to continue my somewhat lonely journey as an interactional sociolinguist working on what is seen by most as a psycholinguistic endeavor.

During my years at the Freie Universität, Berlin, both as a graduate student in the Germanistik Department and later as a *Lehrbeauftragte* teaching at the John F. Kennedy Institut für Nordamerikastudien, I learned a great deal from discussions with Dr. Norbert Dittmar, Dr. Carol Pfaff, Dr. Gisela Klann-Delius, Dr. Jürgen Streeck, Anjuli Gupta, and Carol Kind.

Since my return to the United States and to Georgetown University, first as a visiting faculty member and subsequently as an assistant professor of linguistics, my thinking has been sharpened through enlightening discussions with a number of individuals working in the fields of language and aging and language in clinical populations. In this context, I would especially like to thank Dr. Loraine Obler, Dr. Mark Luborsky, Dr. Bonnie Podraza, and Ms. Marcia Bond. For their support and welcoming spirit, I cannot sufficiently thank the faculty members of the Georgetown Linguistics Department and Dean James E. Alatis of the Georgetown School of Languages and Linguistics. I cannot imagine being happier teaching discourse analysis anywhere else. I especially owe a great debt to Dr. Ralph Fasold for his unending support and encouragement over the past three years. I have learned much from discussions with students in my courses, especially those in my classes on Discourse and Aging, and Discourse in Clinical Populations.

For their able assistance and flexibility, I would like to thank the editors of Cambridge University Press, especially Marion Smith, Judith Ayling, Catherine Max, and Christine Lyall-Grant. Three anonymous reviewers for the Press made a number of insightful comments which led to improvements in both the shape and substance of the manuscript. I am grateful for their careful reading of my words.

Writing a book is a very personal as well as an academic endeavor. Here I would like to thank my family for the important role which they played in helping me to achieve this goal. As far back as I can remember, my parents, Gerald and Claire Ehernberger, encouraged me to set high goals for myself and then had the patience to show me how I might reach those goals. Throughout this project, I have enjoyed the complete support of my best friend and husband, Dan. His own intellectual curiosity and love of new challenges help to bring a sense of balance and sanity to life. Special thanks to my daughter, Siri Liv, whose laughter and tears keep reminding me about what is important.

My heartfelt appreciation goes to Ms. Jill Bergen, former Coordinator of Volunteer Services, The Hermitage in Northern Virginia, for teaching me so much about the institutionalized elderly. My work with her was very rewarding.

And, finally, thank you, "Elsie." My life will forever be enriched by the time we spent together. God bless you.

1   Introduction

Alzheimer's disease is a degenerative brain disease which has major social consequences for the individual who has the disease as well as for those people who are emotionally and/or physically close to this individual. The role which language plays in this relationship stands at the center of the present study. As a complement to traditional analyses of language and Alzheimer's disease based on speech samples elicited in clinical settings, we will examine language in the life of one elderly female Alzheimer's patient, Elsie, from an interactional sociolinguistic perspective. Here the language of our conversations over four-and-one-half years will be investigated both as a changing symptom of the progression of her disease and in my reactions to Elsie's communicative breakdowns and successes. I will attempt to paint a picture of Elsie which goes beyond a mere producer and recipient of the utterances which are the source of the frameworks and findings discussed in this study. I hope the reader will come to know a person with wishes, needs, and intentions, who laughs, gets embarrassed, expresses happiness, confidence, and confusion, and shows love and concern for others – an individual who is both hindered and helped by her conversational partner to succeed in interaction. Elsie's language reflects the mental disability of Alzheimer's disease and holds in it countless secrets regarding her abilities and disabilities. The upcoming analyses and interpretations of Elsie's language use are meant to help us get closer to an understanding of how these abilities and disabilities are related to each other and how they change over time.

Approach

Coupland, Coupland, and Giles (1991: 4) argue that there is "an obligation upon *socially* based research to redress the balance and move away from the cognitive and psycholinguistic concerns that have come to dominate the literatures." Although they are speaking about the field of language and aging in general, I share their frustration with the research imbalance in one area of that large field, namely that of the complex relationships between language and Alzheimer's disease. Most work in this area is being carried out by psycholinguists, neurolinguists, and speech pathologists. And as Widdowson (1988, cited in Tannen 1989: 7) points out, conventions of a paradigm determine not only which topics are worth pursuing, but also the "approved" manner in dealing with them, including such considerations as what counts as data.

The primary approach taken in this study is that of interactional sociolinguistics. This means that readers from fields more typically associated with research on Alzheimer's disease may feel some pangs of culture shock as they make their way through it. This culture shock may have to do with the type of language data used, the elicitation (or, more appropriately, lack thereof) of the data, and the focus on the entire interaction, including the incorporation of a variety of contextual features into the analysis. I will now take up each of these issues in turn.

In this study, I examine the language used in *conversational discourse* rather than primarily word- and sentence-level language. Thanks to a concentration of research over the past decade or so, we now have a firm foundation of knowledge regarding Alzheimer's patients' abilities to recognize and recall lexical items and to carry out syntactic and semantic corrections on sentences in isolation. However, since utterances produced by Alzheimer's patients are generally well formed syntactically, most of them would not appear out of the ordinary in isolation. It is only when they are heard within their communicative context in the pursuit of some interactional goal that they point to a problem. In example 1, the utterances "You can do that. That's a good idea," which are produced by Elsie, are perfectly well formed syntactically and semantically, but become marked in the larger discourse.

Example 1

> ELSIE: And where did you say your home was?
> HEIDI: I'm on Walter Road.
> → ELSIE: You can do that. That's a good idea.

Over the past several years there has been a significant increase in the number of investigations into discourse-level language use by Alzheimer's patients. The bulk of this work, however, focuses not on conversation, but on other types of discourse, such as interviews, narratives, descriptions, and procedural discourse. This recent trend to examine language use across utterances is heartening, because it is critical to the understanding of the inappropriate or irrelevant utterances characteristic of the language used by Alzheimer's patients. To my knowledge, however, the present study represents the first in-depth investigation of how one Alzheimer's patient performs in everyday conversation as her disease progresses and how that performance both influences and is influenced by the behavior of her conversational partner.

Bayles and Kaszniak (1987) recommend systematic study of the conversational ability of dementia patients,[1] because they believe that the loss of such ability is likely to be an early marker of the dementia syndrome. They cite a number of anecdotal reports by researchers and clinicians of such patients having difficulty maintaining conversational topics, being insensitive to others in the conversation, saying either too much or too little, and failing to repair misunderstandings. Bayles and Kaszniak (1987:175) argue that the study of conversation in particular will help researchers find out how patients behave in everyday life because these interactions are "the most naturally occurring linguistic activities." Not all conversations, however, are equally "naturally occurring." This observation leads me to my next point.

The conversational data in this study come from open-ended, *natural* talks with an Alzheimer's patient rather than from speech elicited as part of an experimental research protocol.[2] Several researchers (de Ajuriaguerra and Tissot 1975; Wertz 1987; Sabat, Wiggs, and Pinizzotto 1984; Murphy 1990) have reported that patients' abilities as observed casually outside the test situation seem to be better than their assessment in clinical tests have indicated them to be. This discrepancy is not suprising and can be traced, I believe, to the following three interrelated factors.

One factor underlying differential language use in the experimental and natural contexts is the power structure. An important characteristic of naturally occurring conversations which is difficult to reproduce in the clinical setting is the relatively *symmetrical* relations between interlocutors. In the conversations at the heart of this study, Elsie and I trade off being the "expert" on topics, and both initiate, maintain, and close topics at will. This stands in stark contrast to the typical asymmetrical test situation, in which the physician, therapist, or researcher is in control of the questioning and in which the patient's comments not to the point of the task at hand may be recorded as irrelevant utterances. The relative symmetry of the naturally occurring conversation can be expected to allow the patient to exhibit a fuller communicative repertoire with a

---

[1] As will be discussed below, Alzheimer's patients comprise the largest subgroup of dementia patients.

[2] Of course, it is important to point out that, although the conversations between Elsie and me meet all of my "naturalness" criteria, they would not have taken place at all had I not been involved. The initiation of the conversations, then, can be seen as somewhat less natural than that of conversations she had during the same time period with other residents and staff of the health care center.

greater degree of self-assuredness than she might be able to in a typical clinical situation.

A second factor underlying this differential language use is the patient's perception of the level of formality in the communicative situation. The patient's language is not a static whole which can be tapped accurately in any context. Studies of linguistic variation carried out over the past twenty-five years have shown that there are no "single-style" speakers (Labov 1972a); i.e. that every "normal" speaker varies his or her speech according to the perceived formality of the situation. If a patient perceives the test situation to be more formal than a naturally occurring conversation, she can be expected to pay more attention to her speech in the test situation, thereby exhibiting a different variety of language. Researchers of linguistic variation, however, argue that the variety of language used when the *least* amount of attention is paid to the subject's speech is the most consistent and systematic variety (see Labov 1972d: 293). Since the diagnostic decision as to whether or not a patient has Alzheimer's disease depends to a large extent on what the patient says and how she says it in a clinical examination (see Campbell-Taylor 1984), it can be argued that we need to attempt to tap into the patient's communicative abilities as exhibited in what she seems to perceive as a relatively informal situation.

A third factor underlying the differential language use is the patient's perception of the particular tasks to be performed in the interaction, as well as her attitudes towards these tasks and her motivation to carry them out. If the patient perceives that the primary goal in the clinical setting is to evaluate her language, and that whenever she talks she is fulfilling tasks as predetermined by the clinician, that patient can be expected to use a different kind of language (which reflects her attitudes and level of motivation) than she would use in a conversation which is perceived to have no particular goal beyond sociability (Simmel 1961), or talk for talk's sake.

The apparent discrepancy between language used in natural conversations and that used in clinical test situations has led some researchers to incorporate a segment into their test batteries in which conversational abilities can be observed (e.g. Blanken, Dittmann, Haas, and Wallesch 1987; Illes 1989; De Santi, Obler, Sabo-Abramson, and Goldberger 1990; Ripich, Vertes, Whitehouse, Fulton, and Ekelman 1991; and Causino, Obler, Knoefel, and Albert, forthcoming). In these portions of the test the examiner tries to make the interaction as carefree and spontaneous as possible. Whether or not the researchers succeed in overcoming the differential performance in experimental and natural settings has to do in part with how well they are able to deal with the interrelated factors discussed above: Are they able to reduce the power asymmetry between participants? Are they able to get the patient to use a relatively informal variety of language? Are they able to get the patient to feel that her language is not being evaluated?[3]

Conversations, no matter where they occur or how natural they are, take place between *at least two* people who share time but not necessarily space.[4] Far too many studies of language disability focus, however, on only *one* of the interlocutors, namely the individual with the disability, ignoring the language used by the "normal" conversational partner and its potential influence on the interaction. Crystal (1984: 55, 107) argues that language handicap[5] is "first and foremost an interactive phenomenon" which "needs to be studied in interactive terms." Researchers who have taken an interactional approach with other populations have made some interesting observations. Sabsay and Platt (1985: 115–116), for example, report that in interactions with mentally retarded adults, strategies used by well-intentioned interlocutors to save the face of their retarded conversational partners (Edgerton 1967 called this phenomenon the "benevolent conspiracy") may in fact have the opposite effect. The use of incessant repetition and reformulation of both questions and answers by "normal" interlocutors may not allow the retarded persons the latitude needed to display the competence they have and may indeed force them into looking more incompetent than they are. In their work on intergenerational talk, Coupland, Coupland, Giles, and Henwood (1988) discuss a similar phenomenon, that of a young interlocutor designing her speech according to her stereotyped *perceptions* of what the elderly interlocutor's comprehension abilities are, resulting in the use of over-careful articulation, simple syntactic structures, familiar vocabulary, and a high level of

---

[3] Of course, these points made here are based on the assumption that we are attempting to find out how effectively Alzheimer's patients can communicate in everyday situations. Ulatowska, Allard, Donnell, Bristow, Hayes, Flower, and North (1988) make the important point that spontaneous language tasks may actually make it harder for the clinician to determine the patient's underlying language deficits because the patient can choose communicative strategies in the naturalistic context to help hide a particular problem.

[4] Telephone conversations, for example, connect spaces not shared by the conversationalists. Conversations are typically spoken, but, given the technologies of interactive electronic-mail and TDD (telecommunications device for the deaf), can also be written.

[5] Crystal uses the term "handicap" where I use the term "disability." My decision to use the term "disability" rather than "handicap" or "impairment" is based on St. Claire's (1989) discussion of Wood and Badley's model of disablement (1978a, 1978b, 1980), which distinguishes between *impairment* as a medical disorder (pathological condition), *disability* as the expression of impairments in terms of deviations from performance norms (physical, psychological, and social tasks, skills, and behaviors), and *handicap* as the disadvantage for a given individual resulting from an impairment or disability. Within this tripartite distinction, the present study deals primarily with performance deviations (i.e., disabilities) and not with their cause or whether they result in disadvantage.

redundancy. In this study, I take into account the role of my linguistic contributions in affecting the conversational interactions between Elsie and me, rather than concentrating solely on Elsie's language use. In order to further contextualize and understand the language produced within our interactions, information regarding the physical and emotional environment of our talks, as well as relevant social concerns, such as stigma and face-maintenance, are also brought into the discussion when relevant.

This study is presented as a first step toward a fuller understanding of the interactional contexts of the communicative disorders which accompany Alzheimer's disease and the factors that influence the way these problems are handled by people who care for Alzheimer's patients. It is hoped that the findings and frameworks discussed in upcoming chapters can be creatively and effectively applied in the continuing investigation of discourse produced in interactions with Alzheimer's patients. It is only by teasing apart the variety of influences underlying communicative strengths and weaknesses in real-life interactions that we may come closer to understanding the extent to which the discourse strategies of healthy conversational partners augment or offset the seemingly relentless decline of these patients' communicative abilities. This understanding, then, may ultimately help us to enable these patients to communicate to the best of their abilities.

Before moving ahead to introduce the women whose conversations are at the heart of this study, we turn first to a general discussion of Alzheimer's disease and a review of previous scholarly work on its linguistic manifestations. The following sections are especially important for readers unfamiliar with the relationships between Alzheimer's disease and language, but even experienced researchers may find the discussion of recent findings on discourse-level language abilities useful as they are integrated into the five components of Schiffrin's (1987) interactive discourse model.

Alzheimer's disease

Alzheimer's disease, which was first described by the German neurologist, Alois Alzheimer (1907), is a condition which results in a gradual, and initially subtle, deterioration of intellectual and eventually physical abilities, including memory and perceptual deficits, change in personality, loss of reasoning capacity, difficulty in maintaining attention, orientation, and learning, and differential language loss (see Bayles and Kaszniak 1987, chapter 1, for an excellent overview). Definitive diagnosis of Alzheimer's disease can be made only by biopsy or autopsy of the patient's brain and the subsequent location of the characteristic, abnormal structures called neuritic (or senile) plaques, consisting of degenerating nerve endings, and neurofibrillary tangles, consisting of thousands of pairs of abnormal, twisted filaments, in specific areas of the brain tissues.[6] (See Sloan 1990a for a helpful discussion of Alzheimer's disease and the brain.) However, because there is at present no cure or treatment for Alzheimer's disease, a diagnosis of exclusion (Terry and Katzman 1983), made by ruling out a wide variety of other possible causes for the condition, including vitamin deficiencies, systemic infections, brain tumors, and severe depression, is usually preferred over the much riskier diagnosis by biopsy. The diagnosis of exclusion makes it difficult to provide an accurate estimate of the number of individuals affected by Alzheimer's disease. Projections from a detailed study of East Boston, Massachusetts (Evans *et al*. 1990) estimate that 2.88 million individuals in the US were affected by Alzheimer's disease in 1980. Projections beyond 1980 based on US census population projections estimate that approximately 3.75 million individuals in the US were affected as of 1990 and that, depending on the rate of population growth, this number will reach between 7.5 and 14.3 million by the year 2050. In a separate study, Katzman (1991) estimated that 4 million US Americans have Alzheimer's disease. Alzheimer's disease is the major cause of dementia, a "condition of chronic progressive deterioration in intellect, personality, and communicative functioning" (Bayles and Kaszniak 1987: 1). Estimates of the percentage of all dementia that is thought to be accounted for by Alzheimer's disease range from 70% (Katzman 1991) to 80–90% (US Office of Technology Assessment 1992), although the dementia syndrome is reported to be associated with over fifty different causes (Bayles and Kaszniak 1987).

The cause of Alzheimer's disease is unknown. Possible candidates include genetic factors, chromosomal abnormalities, slow-acting or dormant viruses, accumulation of environmental toxins, such as aluminium, or a combination of the above (Reisberg 1981; Katzman 1985). Bowen (1987) proposes a conceptual model based on Boolean logic to accommodate a multi-factored cause. The key component of this model is an AND gate, which can have any number of inputs and a single output. A particular event turns "on" and remains "on" at its respective input gate. As soon as the necessary number of inputs have been turned "on", the output is realized. In the case of Alzheimer's disease, it is proposed that several factors (as mentioned above) must be present in the life course of

---

[6] At a symposium on "Alzheimer's Disease: The State of Science" organized by the National Institute on Aging at the 1991 Annual Meeting of the Gerontological Society of America in San Francisco, California, Terry (1991) argued that the loss of synapses, especially in the midfrontal region of the brain, is more significant than the presence of either plaques or tangles.

the patient for the degenerative processes to be initiated. Because of this uncertainty in neuropathological research regarding the cause of Alzheimer's disease, Kitwood (1988) argues that inquiry into factors of a more personal nature, such as an individual's psychology and social setting, should not be excluded a priori.

While Alzheimer's disease is not an inevitable part of aging, its incidence does increase with age. To illustrate, Evans *et al.* (1990) estimate that approximately 11.3% of the US population 65 years of age and older are affected by Alzheimer's disease. When one breaks the one age group into three, this trend becomes evident. Of the group 65–74 years of age, it is thought that 3.9% are affected by Alzheimer's disease; of the group 75–84, 16.4% are estimated to be affected; of the group 85 years of age and older, 47.55% are believed to be affected. Some researchers have noted the similarities of behaviors typical of Alzheimer's patients with those of healthy elderly individuals, and have hypothesized that Alzheimer's disease may represent an accelerated version of the normal aging pattern (see Emery 1988: 236 and Ulatowska, Allard, Donnell, Bristow, Hayes, Flower, and North 1988). It is important in this regard to note here that there appear to be only quantitative differences regarding the presence of plaques and tangles in the brains of healthy elderly and those with behavioral signs of Alzheimer's disease. In her report of a conference session examining the relationship of normal aging and dementing diseases of the elderly, Storandt (1987: 1) suggests that any distinction between normal and diseased will be arbitrary because it is based on a cutoff along a continuum that could be placed at numerous points. There is no discrete point at which people necessarily move from health to disability as the disease model implies (see also Kitwood 1988 and Opit 1988 for similar discussions). Katzman (1991) reports that a small percentage of individuals who did not show evidence of Alzheimer's disease while alive have enough tangles and plaques in the autopsy to be classified as having had Alzheimer's disease. This hypothesis of accelerated aging raises the question as to whether or not some of the behaviors exhibited by Alzheimer's patients may partly be the effect of normal aging. The problem as articulated by Sandson, Obler, and Albert (1987) is the difficulty in getting normative data on language behavior of normal, healthy elderly individuals, since this population is always compared to younger people. The result is that we do not know whether and to what extent Alzheimer's behavior may be somewhat inflated by a normal deterioration of some kinds of language use in aging.

When a person is diagnosed as having Alzheimer's disease, or perhaps when his or her family or friends determine that their loved one is becoming "senile", there is a good chance that person will be moved to a nursing home.[7] It is estimated that, at any one time, Alzheimer's patients comprise nearly half of the nursing home population (National Center for Health Statistics 1985, Agency for Health Care Policy and Research 1987) in the US, even though, as noted above (Evans *et al.* 1990), they make up only approximately 11% of the general population 65 years of age and older. It is projected that nearly all Alzheimer's patients will spend some time in a nursing home at some point in their life, according to a report of the US Office of Technology Assessment (1992).

The time an Alzheimer's patient spends in a nursing home may change the way she conceives of herself. Goffman (1961: 12) argues that nursing homes, as well as other kinds of what he terms "total institutions," are "forcing houses for changing persons; each is a natural experiment on what can be done to the self." Such "total institutions" control the whole life and around-the-clock activity of an individual and are characterized by a small supervisory staff who are socially integrated into the outside world managing a large group of live-ins who have restricted contact with the outside. Goffman notes that within a total institution the barriers normally separating sleep, play, and work areas in life are broken down. This altered self-concept may, of course, be coupled with the fact that in many cases the person entering the nursing home already has doubts about her self, in that she is either in a sick role (Parsons 1951) or is questioning her mental health, both of which are considered deviant roles in our society.

In her ethnography of a nursing home, Smithers (1977) offers an insightful portrayal of staff beliefs about senile patients at that institution. She maintains that "in coming to be viewed as senile, patients are judged incapable of functioning rationally and assume a less than human aspect." Additionally, such patients are freed from usual expectations of more rational patients and therefore take on a "non-person" status. This status has potentially serious consequences for staff–patient communication, which in her study rarely extends beyond a few formulaic exchanges, and is not unusual in light of work done on stigmatization. Katz (1981) explains this behavior by pointing out that such contact may remind the normal person of his vulnerability to sudden misfortune, or raise the prospect of becoming enmeshed in another person's dependency.

In her in-depth investigation into communicative opportunities in nursing homes, Lubinski (1981) suggests, too, that the problem and the

---

[7] This discussion on nursing homes is not meant to denigrate nursing homes, nor is it meant to cause relatives of Alzheimer's patients to feel guilty if they have placed their loved one in such an institution. There are many fine nursing homes, including the one where the conversations investigated in this study took place. Because of the steadily increasing amount of care needed by Alzheimer's patients as the disease progresses, moving them into a nursing home is often an unavoidable step.

solution may be intertwined. She notes that, since people find it difficult to talk with patients with specific communication problems and more general cognitive disorders, these patients have decreased opportunities to communicate meaningfully. This situation may result in the gradual withdrawal from opportunities that actually are available because the patient may think it is easier to remain silent than to face the problems and frustrations of communicating.

The communicative difficulties associated with Alzheimer's disease contribute heavily to the stigma which is associated with the disease. Goffman (1963) and Katz (1981) suggest that stigmas related to speech or communication are worse than physical stigmas which can more easily be concealed: the communicative stigmas are made obvious each time the individual opens his or her mouth to speak. These communicative difficulties increase the tension found in virtually all conversations between getting information across and saving face as the healthy conversational partners try *not* to draw attention to the problems caused by the cognitive disability in the interaction.

Based on her own experiences as a nurses' aid in a nursing home, Rust (1986: 138, 140) provides a personal account of how the factors just discussed affect the life of one 83-year-old woman, Amy, who was diagnosed as having senile dementia:

Her life is considered to be over and because of this she is not perceived or treated as creative, adaptive, engaged – all the attributes of being human and alive. Instead, she barely exists in a limbo of invisibility where her body, her self, and her expression are not considered her own . . . Talking is Amy's way of knowing she is still alive. It is her intense, continuous engagement. It is one of the very means of creative expression allowed her. It is a way of creatively adapting to a monotonous and inhuman environment where no one really talks with her. If she stops talking, she'll "just stop."

Rust goes on to echo the suggestion made above that the problem and the solution may indeed be intertwined. She speculates that many of the symptoms of dementia, such as confusion, withdrawal, hostility, and repeated phrases, may be, in part, a reaction to the lack of "genuine, egalitarian" communicative opportunities in the institution.

But even if the Alzheimer's patient is not in a nursing home, her communicative opportunities may still be reduced in quantity or in quality. Williams and Giles (1991) point out that negative stereotyping (which may result from communicative difficulties, for example) on the part of actual or potential conversational partners, can have personal consequences for the patient, such as diminished opportunities to be treated as an individual with individual needs and desires, or the diminished opportunities for talk and social interaction discussed above.

With this general overview of Alzheimer's disease as a backdrop, we now focus in specifically on how language relates to the overall picture just outlined. Following a more global discussion of the communicative difficulties of Alzheimer's patients, specific findings in the areas of word-finding difficulties and discourse-level behavior are presented.

Linguistic analyses of Alzheimer's disease

One manifestation of Alzheimer's disease is a progressive and apparently irreversible deterioration of the patient's ability to communicate with others. The patient may have trouble finding the appropriate word in a conversation. She may have trouble tracking and using pronouns appropriately or in understanding indirectness as it was intended. On the other hand, she may continue to be able to carry out some of the more mechanical tasks in interaction, such as taking a turn-at-talk or getting someone's attention. She may even perform better if dealing with a topic of personal importance rather than a more banal one.

Based on their own observations of the use of language by Alzheimer's patients as well as on those of other researchers, Bayles (1984), Obler and Albert (1984), and Overman and Geoffrey (1987) offer the following characterization of three basic stages of the disease in terms of communicative decline. These researchers note that this characterization is based on the findings of a variety of synchronic studies of patients at various stages of the disease. It is, therefore, somewhat artificial, and should remain somewhat tentative until it can be corroborated by longitudinal studies of patients' communicative behavior over time. The *early or mild stage* of Alzheimer's disease is marked primarily by memory problems. Subtle language problems, such as object-naming difficulty, may be masked by strategies developed by the patient. The patient may be disoriented for time, but generally not for place or person. The discourse may be somewhat wordy, imprecise, and off-topic. Sarcasm and humor may be difficult for the patient to detect. In the *middle or moderate stage*, naming problems become more marked, conversation seems devoid of meaning, often irrelevant, and somewhat less interactive in nature. The patient is disoriented for time and place, but not for self, and seems to have comprehension difficulties. In the *late or severe stage*, the patient is disoriented for time, place, and person. There is a general lack of communication and possibly even lack of awareness that another person is present. The limited discourse that is produced is filled with repetition, jargon, and bizarre, nonsensical utterances. Syntax and phonology may finally become somewhat disrupted after having remained intact until this stage of the illness. In the very final stages, language may become personal and idiosyncratic (Emery 1988), and possibly echolalic, before the patient becomes mute.

It is generally agreed that, at least up until the final stage of the disease, Alzheimer's patients' problems in communication are due less to phonological and morphosyntactic disorders than to difficulties on the semantic and pragmatic levels (Bayles 1979; Schwartz, Marin, and Saffran 1979; Obler 1981; Appell, Kertesz, and Fisman 1982; Kempler 1984; Bayles 1985; Bayles and Kaszniak 1987; Smith, Chenery, and Murdoch 1989; Ulatowska, Allard, and Chapman 1990). The characterization by Appell, Kertesz, and Fisman (1982: 83) of the spontaneous speech of their Alzheimer's patient as "fluent irrelevant speech, with well-preserved syntax and words, yet for practical purposes the meaning is lost" is typical. Kempler (1984) determined that Alzheimer's patients not only have a good command of syntax, but appear to use approximately the same level of syntactic complexity as healthy age-matched individuals. This finding is important, because it might be argued that Alzheimer's patients only appear to have a good command of syntax by overusing simpler structures. As Kempler maintains, his results extend the characterization of Alzheimer's speech from *fluent* to *syntactically normal*.

Word-finding difficulties

A great deal of attention has been directed at the word-finding difficulties as mentioned above in the characterization of the communicative decline which accompanies Alzheimer's disease.[8] This situation is probably due in large part to the fact that such word-finding difficulties occur early and frequently in the progression of the disease and are relatively easy to identify. These factors make this phenomenon well suited to experimental testing (Irigaray 1973; Gardner 1974; Schwartz, Marin, and Saffran 1979; Bayles 1979, 1982; Obler 1981; Appell, Kertesz, and Fisman 1982; Martin and Fedio 1983; Kempler 1984; Nebes, Martin, and Horn 1984; Hier, Hagenlocker, and Shindler 1985; Huff, Corkin, and Growdon 1986; Flicker, Ferris, Crook, and Bartus 1987; Murdoch, Chenery, Wilks, and Boyle 1987; Sandson, Obler, and Albert 1987; Huff, Mack, Mahlmann, and Greenberg 1988; and Shuttleworth and Huber 1988).

As could be expected, researchers have focused on a variety of questions

---

[8] Obler and Albert (1980a) maintain that the word-finding difficulties which are characteristic of Alzheimer's patients are also found, although to a lesser extent, in the healthy elderly. The difference lies, according to Obler and Albert, in the type of response these two populations provide to their disability. The healthy elderly cue themselves into the right word by providing an appropriate syntactic context; Alzheimer's patients, on the other hand, either provide a substitute word or give up the task.

which help us to systematize the relevant findings. Possibly the most basic question has to do with determining whether a patient's word-finding difficulty is simply an artifact of the test situation, i.e., that the patient is indeed capable of finding words but not in a test situation. Nebes, Martin, and Horn (1984) support the idea that the semantic memory is not disrupted at all; they blame the large amount of attention that patients have to pay to carry out the task-at-hand in the test situation for their poor performance. Blanken, Dittmann, Haas, and Wallesch (1987) support this viewpoint, in that they found no significant difference in word-finding ability in spontaneous speech (in response to an interviewer's open-ended questions) from that of controls.

Although it may be true that word-finding difficulties are exaggerated or highlighted in test situations as compared with spontaneous speech, other research involving conversational speech components (including the present study) indicate the prominence of word-finding difficulties across the span of the disease. Such considerations of the influence of the eliciting context on specific communicative phenomena are important, however, because they highlight the question of relative automatic versus effortful processing. Where a process is more automatic, such as is provided in a natural setting, the patient can be expected to do better than in situations where the process is more effortful, such as in a test situation. Even within the test situation, Huff, Corkin, and Growdon (1986) discovered that the relative amount of effort required to complete a naming task played a role in the patients' level of performance. In the relatively effortful test of category fluency, where patients are asked to list aloud as many words within a category (such as vehicles, vegetables, tools, and clothing) as they can within a one-minute time period, the difference in performance level between the Alzheimer's patients and the control group in the study was much greater than for the relatively more automatic test of confrontation naming, in which patients are shown line drawings of objects from the categories used in the fluency test and are allowed 30 seconds to name each object.

Another more difficult question gets at the heart of the issue of language problems and Alzheimer's disease in general, that is, whether the naming difficulty represents an actual lexical semantic loss or more simply an access problem. Nebes (1985) and Sandson, Obler, and Albert (1987) suggest that semantic memory is preserved in dementia; the problem is an impairment in access, especially in the kind of effortful active search of semantic memory we discussed above. Evidence for the preservation of semantic memory comes from the fact that phonological cues often seem to assist the patient in retrieving the word in question. Some tentative support for the lexical loss hypothesis, on the other hand, is provided by

Henderson, Mack, Freed, Kempler, and Anderson (1990), who found that 80% of the errors on the Boston Naming Test (Kaplan, Goodglass, and Weintraub 1983) were consistent in two administrations of the examination six months apart. Henderson *et al.* argue that a problem of lexical access implies variable word-finding difficulty; a theory of lexical loss predicts that many lexical items would be consistently unavailable, as seemed to be the case in their study. The researchers advise some caution in the matter, however, since some patients actually performed better on the second administration of the naming test.

Whatever the underlying cause of the word-finding difficulty, the manifestations of this problem in the patient's production of discourse are varied. Most characteristic appears to be the use of an imprecise substitute, such as *thing* for *match*, or a word which is semantically related to but not a synonym of the "lost" word, such as *truck* for *locomotive*. Other manifestations are circumlocutions (descriptions of the target word without using it), such as *a thing you light cigarettes with* for *match*, and phonetic or semantic paraphasias (mispronunciation or choosing of the wrong word), such as *colmotive* for *locomotive* or *firebug* for *match* (examples of paraphasias drawn from Appell, Kertesz, and Fisman 1982). Bayles (1985) suggests that semantic features appear to be lost progressively, with mistakes at first seeming to be related semantically to the stimulus item and becoming less logical as the disease progresses. In Kempler's (1984) examination of word-finding difficulties in a confrontation naming test, he found that the majority of the errors (66%) made by the patients were semantically related to the target object. These semantically related answers fell into the following five categories: functional description (*for fishing* for *rowboat*), part–whole relationship (*house* for *window*), novel form (*salt holder* for *salt shaker*), substitution of a hyponym (*moon* for *sun*), and physical description (*it has a glitter to it* for *sun*). When the same patients were telling him about their family within more conversational discourse, Kempler observed that word-finding errors always preserved form class (verbs for verbs, nouns for nouns, etc.) and that many were semantically related to the supposed target word (*son* for *father*, *spelling* for *pronunciation*). He also found an excessive use of pronouns and empty words by the patients. The high incidence of imprecise words like *thing* and *place* instead of more meaningful substantives leads Alzheimer's discourse to be characterized as "empty" and is the reason behind many of the understanding problems listeners experience in conversations with these patients. This increased use of "empty" words and pronouns has been noted by others, including Hier, Hagenlocker, and Shindler (1985), Bayles, Tomoeda, Kaszniak, Sterns, and Eagans (1985),

Nicholas, Obler, Albert, and Helm-Estabrooks (1985), and Sandson, Obler, and Albert (1987).

Bayles (1979: 110) found that, in addition to the large number of semantically related responses, there were also many responses which were "not obviously related to the test item" and illustrates this observation with the following examples: *country folks* for *flag*, *where is the baby?* for *matches*, and *they're pretty* for *flowers*. If we use as a working hypothesis that these patients perform better on emotional topics than on mundane topics (see discussion in Boller, Cole, Vrtunski, Patterson, and Kim 1979: 164), however, we can come up with likely scenarios which produced the responses above. For example, seeing a picture of matches may have aroused the protective feeling of a caregiver attempting to keep matches away from a baby. Seeing a picture of a flag may have stirred up memories or stereotypes in the patient of "country folks" involved in patriotic festivities. Seeing a picture of flowers apparently elicited an emotional, evaluative response of *they're pretty* rather than the requested lexical item *flowers*. Evidence of Alzheimer's patients responding in a personal way to an impersonal task is also observed in segments of the test battery other than naming tests. Bayles (1984) shares with us the response of one Alzheimer's patient to the task of describing a marble. Included in his response to "Tell me about this" is the personal commentary: "It's not mine. I didn't have it." Emery (1988: 235) notes that three of the twenty patients in her study "interjected highly personal meaning into the context, demonstrating an inability to share in normative connotation." In response to a command to point to a blue circle in the test situation, one patient pointed to the circles under her eyes. In another situation, a patient responded to the question "Who is president?" with the following personal commentary: "Well, it isn't me . . . it's the one who was straight up."

These clinical observations bring to mind Rosen's (1988) discussion of the autobiographical impulse which he maintains is a constant factor in human discourse. He speaks of the "clandestine presence of memory" and suggests that "in the process of the construction of many kinds of texts, spoken and written, the memories of the past are in constant play flashing beneath the still surface like gleaming fish in a still lake." These data suggest that word-finding problems of Alzheimer's patients tell us not only about relationships between words at the level of semantic features, but may indicate that word meaning is tied in with personal experiences. Further study along these lines could have important implications for work on semantic and episodic memory, as discussed by Tulving (1972), semantic memory being knowledge of words and episodic meaning referring to memory for specific events in time. Clark (1980: 56) states that "information stored in the semantic system must have entered the system during some period of episodic learning ... Conversely, episodic memories are built from information in semantic memory." Could it be that in some cases of word-finding difficulty, the patient is denied direct access to semantic memory and is detoured through episodic memory, resulting in a response seemingly unrelated to the test item? Because episodic memory is experientially based and is therefore much more individual than semantic memory, the patient's response may indeed *not* be unrelated to the test item; it only *appears* to be unrelated because we do not share information which is in the patient's episodic memory.

Regardless of the answers to the questions above, the difficulty in finding words has real-life implications for the patients with this problem. Because this common word-finding difficulty detracts significantly from the patients' ability to communicate and, consequently, from their capacity to interact socially and function independently, Flicker, Ferris, Crook, and Bartus (1987: 198) emphasize the relevance of the object-naming task to the diagnosis of Alzheimer's disease and to the measurement of any therapeutic success with this population. These word-finding difficulties that Alzheimer's patients experience manifest themselves in a variety of ways in natural conversation. Contrasted with problems on the naming tasks in a test situation, word-finding problems may not be immediately obvious to other participants in natural conversations. A circumlocution may seem to a listener like a somewhat "roundabout" way of talking but may not impede understanding. A vague or "empty" word may shift the burden of sense-making in the conversation to the listener, who may or may not be able to reach an adequate understanding of the discourse. A semantically related word may provide just enough clues to the listener (especially if additional clues can come from the physical environment) to allow adequate understanding, although initially this related but unintended word may cause the conversational partner some confusion. A mischosen word, such as "dress" for "painting" (as discussed in chapter 2) may cause the interlocutor severe confusion which may be alleviated only by additional clues from the physical suroundings. Similarly, the use of a newly coined word will most certainly be problematic for the listener. Assuming that these alternative displays of word-finding difficulties are incorporated into syntactically correct utterances, as has been observed to be the case in study after study with Alzheimer's patients, the utterances will be alternatively judged to be (1) fine semantically, although somewhat wordy (in the case of circumlocutions), (2) fine semantically, although the listener may come away with an interpretation other than the one intended by the speaker (as in some cases of mischosen words and semantically related words, (3) odd semantically on the sentence level (as in some cases of mischosen words or semantically related words), or (4) odd semantically on the lexical level (as in the case of neologisms).

Discourse-level difficulties

Compared with the amount of research on the word-finding difficulties of Alzheimer's patients, relatively little attention has been directed at analyzing discourse-level problems. Most studies of Alzheimer's patients' linguistic (dis)abilities to date have involved test situations in which the patients perform various tasks (e.g. naming objects in photographs or drawings, performing transformations on sentences, and disambiguating spoken homophones). As mentioned above, this situation has begun to change over recent years, but even today, studies which focus on discourse are carried out almost exclusively within an experimental paradigm.

When a "spontaneous" speech component has been included in the overall study, it has frequently been in the form of discourse elicited by a request from the researcher for the patient to talk about a specific topic. For example, in Irigaray's (1973) study, seven of her thirty-two subjects were encouraged to talk about the course of their illness, their profession, and their families. In their study of patterns of discourse cohesion and coherence in Alzheimer's disease, Ripich and Terrell (1988) based their findings on speech samples of "topic-directed interviews" in which three topics – family, daily activities, and health – were introduced by the researcher through open-ended questions. Although Ripich and Terrell characterize the resulting discourse as "a natural flow of interaction between the subject and the interviewer," one cannot help but note the lack of symmetry in the discourse in terms of control of topic. In Kempler's (1984) study of the syntactic, semantic, and pantomime abilities of Alzheimer's patients, he collected two "spontaneous" language samples, one being a biographical interview and the other a narrative description of the Cookie Theft Picture from the Boston Diagnostic Aphasia Examination (Goodglass and Kaplan 1972). In Bayles' studies (1979, 1982) "the only test requiring subjects to use speech *creatively*" (1979: 134) (my emphasis) was a test called the "Verbal Expression Test." In this test, which was modeled after a subtest of the Illinois Test of Psycholinguistic Abilities, patients are given an envelope, a button, a nail, and a marble and are "instructed to tell everything they could about them" (1979: 72). Example 2 illustrates the type of discourse which results from talking about a button:

Example 2

E: Tell me everything you can about this.
(button)
P: It's a button, a large button with two little holes in it.
(extended pause)
E: Can you tell me any more about it?
P: Well, not much. It's just two little holes in the button. I'd have
to say it fast with two little holes in it.

(Bayles 1982: 275)

Bayles' (1979) observation that "the patient did not seem capable of calling to mind much that could be said about the button in spite of the urgings of the examiner" may in fact be valid. However, this may be not so much a case of disability but rather unwillingness to respond. It is possible that the patient sees no need to elaborate on a button. Thus, it is not surprising that patients' strategies observed by Bayles in response to such topics included stating that the "task asked of them was trivial and should be dismissed" or repeating what they had already said as "a common means of trying to make what was said seem like more" (Bayles 1982: 275). Bayles interprets these responses as examples of "strategies to conceal their [the patients'] deficiencies." Again, it may very well be the case that these are examples of such concealment strategies. On the other hand, regarding the first type of response, it *is* true that the task *is* trivial and the patient's response is, therefore, completely appropriate. The fact that healthy subjects usually comply with this type of request may indicate greater understanding and/or acceptance of artificial test situations, where the *need* to communicate is not clear. Regarding the second type of response, it would not be surprising if even healthy subjects tended to repeat their answer to such a test question in their attempt to balance the fact that there is not much that can be said about a button with the expectation in a test situation that a lengthy response must be provided.

The danger here is that many descriptions in the literature of the discourse abilities of Alzheimer's patients seem to be based on limited data in response to limited topics, and may not be completely valid for a great deal of Alzheimer's discourse. For example, Obler (1981: 380) in her review of Irigaray (1973) states: "Indeed the abilities to initiate speech, to maintain speech, and to appropriately stop speech, taken for granted in normals, may all be impaired in the language of dementing individuals." Furthermore, she observes that Irigaray's conversational data show that "second person pronouns simply do not occur in dementing speech, nor do questions or commands" in addition to the "lack of either modificatory comments on the truth values of the patient's statement (*maybe, undoubtedly*) or the lack of reference to speaker as ego (e.g., *I think, I believe*)" (Obler 1981: 382).

In response to Obler's remarks above, Appell, Kertesz, and Fisman (1982: 76) observe: "All reflect the breakdowns of language as a tool: for communicating with others, for conveying or obtaining information, for directing actions, either of oneself or of others, for generating concepts about the world and forming propositions about it, and for testing the truth of such propositions and drawing implications from them." When one looks at the small portions of transcript reproduced in Bayles (1979, 1982) or Kempler (1984) and the discourse described and analyzed in the present study, however, the remarks above appear *either* to describe only later stages in the progression of the disease *or* perhaps talk within a limited experimental setting, in which even the "spontaneous" talk is in fact elicited by interview questions. When these patients are not observed in a natural setting which allows them to speak at their own pace about their own topics, it is not surprising that they are found to be unable to use language "as a tool: for communicating with others" (Appell, Kertesz, and Fisman 1982: 76). Any resulting conclusions regarding their ability to use language creatively to communicate should be carefully considered. Could it be that these conclusions are just describing the limited amount of communication in the testing situation? There must be a need for the patient to communicate before we can be sure that our statements regarding that patient's ability to communicate are valid.

Given the relatively large amount of work in recent years on various genres of Alzheimer's patients' discourse, including narratives, descriptions, procedural discourse, interviews, and more-or-less conversational discourse, it seems to me to be useful to discuss the studies and their findings with reference to Schiffrin's (1987) model of discourse. Briefly summarized, Schiffrin's interactive model has five components which work together to create local coherence: (1) an exchange structure; (2) an action structure; (3) an ideational structure; (4) an information state; and (5) a participant framework. Schiffrin (1987: 29) defines local coherence in discourse as "the outcome of joint efforts from interactants to *integrate* knowing, meaning, saying and doing." Each of the five components will be discussed in turn with specific reference to the relevant research findings regarding Alzheimer's disease and language.

Exchange structure

By "exchange structure," Schiffrin is referring to those discourse phenomena which fulfill the mechanical requirements of talk, such as turns-at-talk and conditionally relevant adjacency pairs (see Sacks, Schegloff, and Jefferson 1978, and Schegloff and Sacks 1973), including such paired phenomena as question/answer, invitation/acceptance, complaint/denial, and greeting/greeting.

Sabat, Wiggs, and Pinizzotto (1984) in their observations of the behavior of two Alzheimer's patients in their homes report that, despite generally incoherent speech, one patient "would pause to give the observer a turn to converse," indicating that the patient could still manage such structural tasks as turn-taking in conversation. This finding is consistent with that reported in Golper and Binder (1981) that conversational turn-taking is maintained in the early and middle stages of Alzheimer's disease. Sabat *et al.* go on to observe, however, that the patient's responses to the observer's questions were not consistently appropriate. In one example, the patient gave a yes-no answer to a wh-question.

Example 3

OBSERVER: How are you feeling?
PATIENT: Yes – and they like it that way.

(Sabat, Wiggs, and Pinizzotto 1984: 346)

In their examination of ten late-stage Alzheimer's patients, Causino, Obler, Knoefel, and Albert (forthcoming) found that turn-taking ability was relatively spared for seven of the subjects. Causino *et al.* point out, however, that in order to obtain responses from patients the researchers often had to give the patients a much longer time to respond than is normally allowed in conversation. Obler (1981) suggests that the phenomenon of silence or "muteness" characteristic of some Alzheimer's patients, besides being associated with the decrease in initiative typical of later stages of the disease, may be further explained as an artifact of long response lags and the "normal" conversational partner not waiting long enough for a response. Sabat (1991) provides further evidence for this explanation in his report on several conversations he had with one Alzheimer's patient. During these conversations he purposefully altered his usual turn-taking behavior in order to give the patient the opportunity to continue what she had been saying before a fairly lengthy pause occurred in the conversation; the patient took advantage of this opportunity. Sabat suggests that had he behaved in his usual way regarding turn-taking, the conversation would have broken down, leaving the patient with a series of incomplete thoughts and the researcher essentially without a partner in the conversation.

Regarding number of utterances and turns, Hutchinson and Jensen (1980) observed that in general the five senile dementia patients in their study produced fewer utterances and more turns than the five elderly controls during three 15-minute segments of conversation, for an end result of noticeably fewer utterances per turn. They interpret this finding as a strategy of limited elaboration which is a result of the patients' assumption that their words convey more meaning than they actually do. Ripich and Terell (1988) also found that the turns produced by the Alzheimer's patients in their study were briefer than those produced by the normal elderly controls. Although the patients produced more than twice as many words as the control group, they produced four times as many turns.

Action structure

By "action structure," Schiffrin is referring to the fact not only that actions are carried out in talk (see Austin 1962 and Searle 1969 for a discussion of speech act theory) but that these actions are situated with regard to previous and subsequent actions.

In their analysis of speech act distribution in the conversational discourse described above, Hutchinson and Jensen (1980) discovered that the senile patients used more directives than the healthy elderly individuals did. These directives were primarily requests for identification, confirmation, and explanation. Many of these requests were made outside of the ongoing topic, exhibiting the patients' sudden shifts in focus to a person or object in the environment (such as asking for information on a fellow patient walking down the hall or an object in the room). The eleven early to midstage Alzheimer's patients in a study carried out by Ripich, Vertes, Whitehouse, Fulton, and Ekelman (1991) also were found to use more requestives (to solicit information or actions) than assertives (to report facts, state rules, and convey attitudes) than the eleven healthy elderly controls during a 9-minute conversation they had with the examiner during a break from testing. Ripich *et al.* interpret this finding as evidence that in the early to middle stages of Alzheimer's disease, patients use requests to help them gain additional information to facilitate their effective participation in the interaction. These findings are in contrast to Bayles' (1984) anecdotal report of a decline in requestives in the middle stages of Alzheimer's disease.

With regard to Alzheimer's patients' abilities to respond to various speech actions, Stevens (1985 as cited in Fromm 1988) reports that significantly more of his fifty subjects were able to respond appropriately to social questions, such as "How are you today?" than to questions asking for information. Fromm and Holland (1989) also report this relative sparing of social convention abilities of the mild and moderate Alzheimer's patients in their study, as compared with their irrelevant, vague, and incomplete responses to requests for information.

A number of researchers have reported that Alzheimer's patients often comment on a required task rather than performing it (Obler 1981; Mace and Rabins 1981; Hier, Hagenlocker, and Shindler 1985; Ulatowska, Allard, Donnell, Bristow, Hayes, Flower, and North 1988). In these cases, the patients may be interpreting the action intended by the examiner (e.g. a request for action on the part of the patient) as another action (e.g. a request for information). This mismatch is interpreted by some researchers as intentional, by others as unintentional. Obler (1981: 382) calls this a "clever strategy, in the event that one expects not to be able to perform correctly" because a comment about the task itself or one's feelings about it cannot really be considered wrong. Mace and Rabins cite the example of a patient who is asked whether he knows the word *wristwatch*.

Example 4

DOCTOR: Do you know what to call this?
PATIENT: Of course I do. Why do you ask?

(Mace and Rabins 1981: 29)

Because he is asked a question about his abilities, the patient is able to respond to the question and avoid the implicit request for the answer (intentional mismatch). Of course, it is possible that the patient has a problem understanding the indirect request for the lexical item (unintentional mismatch), and is responding merely to the directly posed question. Along this line, Appell, Kertesz, and Fisman (1982) note the difficulty on the part of the patient in their case study in drawing inferences.

Ideational structure

By "ideational structure" Schiffrin is referring to the propositions, or what she terms "ideas," in discourse. In this discussion, Schiffrin points out three different relations which hold between ideas. These are (1) cohesive relations (see Halliday and Hasan 1976), (2) topic relations (see Brown and Yule 1983, chapter 3), and (3) functional relations, as illustrated by the relationship between two propositions in a narrative, one providing background information and the other providing information regarding actions (orientation clause and complicating action clause, respectively, according to Labov's (1972b) classic treatment of conversational narratives).

Ripich and Terrell (1988) found no significant differences in the proportionate use of what they call complete propositions, incomplete propositions, and non-propositions by six Alzheimer's patients and six normal elderly controls. In contrast, Ulatowska, Allard, Donnell, Bristow, Hayes, Flower, and North (1988) reported that the Alzheimer's patients in their study conveyed fewer propositions in the course of telling a story, even though they produced as much language as the control group. The patients produced many metalinguistic comments which were viewed as irrelevant propositions within the designated task.

With regard to cohesive ties, Shekim (1983) found that her group of nine Alzheimer's patients at different stages of the disease used significantly fewer cohesive ties per 'communication unit' than did the nine subjects comprising the control group across all discourse types (including narrative, expository, and procedural discourse). Ripich and Terrell (1988) provide further evidence for this finding by observing that cohesion was "disrupted" more than twice as frequently for the Alzheimer's group as for the elderly comparison group in their study. The primary difficulty was the absence of a necessary referent.

Regarding topic control, Hutchinson and Jensen (1980) found that the senile patients in their study initiated new topics much more frequently than the healthy control group did, with many of these introductions coming in the absence of appropriate closing of the current topic. Example 5 illustrates this kind of inappropriate topic initiation.

Example 5

    s: And she was my horse and I would harness her and hitch her up. I would always pat her and smooth her hair and pet her so she'd like me. I didn't want her to be afraid that I'd hurt her, but I never did. She was a nice horse. We liked her.

    E: Did you train her?

  > s: Well, my flowers you folks brought me today ... Aren't they beautiful?

(Hutchinson and Jensen 1980: 69)

Here, instead of answering the question about training her horse, the patient changes the subject to the flowers which her visitors brought. Campbell-Taylor (1984) reports that inappropriate topic shifts were identified by both professional clinicians and non-professionals as characteristic of the oral discourse of one Alzheimer's patient based on a videotape of that patient conversing with a clinician.

In a rare examination of conversations among Alzheimer's patients,

Smith and Ventis (1990) observed that topic development occurred less frequently in conversations among these patients than in conversations between patients and healthy interlocutors. When it did occur, however, Smith and Ventis argue that it was in a "more tolerant and flexible fashion," allowing ambiguous topics, ficticious topics, and what they term "stretched connections." Example 6 illustrates this tolerance.

> *Example 6*
>
> PATIENT 1: Yahal.
> PATIENT 2: Umm hmm. Looks like it's gonna rain too.
> PATIENT 1: Yeah.
>
> (Smith and Ventis 1990: 10)

Closely related to difficulties with topic is the phenomenon of ideational perseveration reported by Bayles, Tomoeda, Kaszniak, Stern, and Eagans (1985). This type of perseveration, i.e. when an idea (rather than a sound, word, or phrase) is expressed more than once and inappropriately to a stimulus, is the most common type of perseveration used by dementia patients. Possible explanations for the phenomenon of perseveration given by Shindler, Caplan, and Hier (1984) include the patient's inability to monitor his or her own speech and the inability to change mental sets. This inability to change mental sets has sometimes been called context-boundedness or stimulus-boundedness in the literature (Obler 1981; Appell, Kertesz, and Fisman 1982) and refers to the patient's reduced ability to free herself from the immediate temporal and spatial context.

In their discussion of the intrusion of tangential or irrelevant information into Alzheimer's patients' narratives and procedural discourse, Ulatowska, Allard, and Chapman (1990) bring up the possibility that this intrusion may reflect a deficit in using story schemas and script knowledge to guide the patients' production of such discourse. However, since Ulatowska and her colleagues found that most of the essential components or steps were actually included in the discourse (suggesting that these underlying structures were relatively intact), they speculate that the intrusion of irrelevant information may instead be a result of memory or attention problems, or a failure on the part of the patients to monitor whether their discourse was clear to the listener.

Grafman, Thompson, Weingartner, Martinez, Lawlor, and Sunderland (1991) investigated Alzheimer's patients' production of such scripts in an attempt to determine whether the breakdown in script production would be like that of the impaired lexical production discussed in the section on word-finding above. Their findings suggest that the internal structure of a script is indeed similar to that of a lexical network, and offer possible reasons underlying Alzheimer's patients' difficulties in producing discourse which relies upon events being reported in a typical sequence.

Information state

By "information state," Schiffrin is referring to the organization and management of knowledge and meta-knowledge (knowledge about knowledge) in the discourse. Can the patient accurately assess the information state of her conversational partner on a particular issue and design her utterance taking that into account? Does the patient seem to know what she does or does not know about a subject?

In their examination of the coherence of discourse as perceived by healthy listeners, Ripich and Terrell (1988) found that information errors accounted for 82% (9 of 11 instances of incoherence) of the perceived incoherence. One of the listeners described the task of following Alzheimer's discourse as "being led across a bridge that suddenly drops into an abyss" (Ripich and Terrell 1988: 14). This difficulty on the part of the listeners seems to be due at least partially to the patients' reduced sensitivity to the needs of their listeners. This notion has been discussed by Hutchinson and Jensen (1980), Richardson and Marquandt (1985), Hamilton (1988, 1991), and Ulatowska, Allard, Donnell, Bristow, Hayes, Flower, and North (1988), and is taken up in some detail in the next chapter.

In their examination of narrative and procedural discourse produced by ten mildly to moderately impaired Alzheimer's patients as compared with ten matched controls, Ulatowska, Allard, and Chapman (1990) observe that the discourse produced by the Alzheimer's subjects was characterized by (1) a reduction of information determined a priori to be essential to each narrative or procedure, (2) an increase in tangential or irrelevant information, and (3) a disruption of reference (inappropriate use of pronouns in the place of nouns).

In comparing 60-second speech samples of early and late Alzheimer's patients describing the Cookie Theft Picture from the Boston Diagnostic Aphasia Examination (Goodglass and Kaplan 1972), Hier, Hagenlocker, and Shindler (1985) reported that the more severely affected patients use no fewer words during the 60 seconds (although an increasing proportion of these words are empty and pro-forms), but make fewer relevant observations, with the result that their speech conveys less information over time.

That Alzheimer's patients' discourse is vague and verbose has been observed and discussed by a variety of researchers (Obler and Albert 1981;

Shekim 1983; Blanken, Dittmann, Haas, and Wallesch 1987; Sandson, Obler, and Albert 1987; Ripich and Terrell 1988). My own research suggests that this is particularly true for the middle stages of the disease. Whereas the initial stages may be somewhat vague, the wordiness increases and compounds the problem in the middle stage. In the final stages of the disease, the vagueness remains, but the wordiness declines in a transition to a mute stage.

Given the dynamic nature of the information state, speakers must be able to continually monitor what they are saying so as to meet the informational needs of the listener(s), and make self-corrections where deemed necessary. Illes (1989) reports that, up to the midstage of the disease, Alzheimer's patients increasingly make use of self-corrections in their responses to open-ended autobiographical questions, indicating an awareness of their own verbal difficulties. The significant increase in the number of aborted phrases at the midstage, however, may reflect the eventual failure of this self-correction strategy. The phenomenon of aborted phrases had been reported earlier by Hier, Hagenlocker, and Shindler (1985) and had been attributed to patients' failure to perceive the necessity to complete their utterances.

In addition to these production-level information difficulties, Alzheimer's patients may also have problems comprehending information. In their examination of responses by ten Alzheimer's patients of moderate severity to 180 questions by an interviewer, Blanken, Dittmann, Haas, and Wallesch (1987) suggest that the problem underlying patients' inappropriate responses has less to do with linguistic production than with information tracking on the part of the patients.

Participant framework

By "participant framework" Schiffrin refers to the relationships between interlocutors in a conversation, as well as to their relationships to what they are saying and doing in the conversations. Does the patient seem to be able to assess accurately her relationship to the interlocutor and to use this assessment to design an utterance or to take a stance toward a particular action? Here it is important to ask who the interlocutors are and what their relationship is to one another. Possible relevant characteristics of the conversational partners are age, sex, ethnic group, level of education, socio-economic status, geographic origin, and so on. Regarding the relationship between the patient and his or her interlocutor, it is important to know the degree to which they know each other, whether they get along with each other, and what the power relationship is.

Ripich, Vertes, Whitehouse, Fulton, and Ekelman (1991: 332) point to the paucity of research done in this interactional area of discourse by observing that, "although the literature reveals little information regarding discourse of SDAT [Alzheimer's] patients, even less is reported about the discourse of their partners. Knowledge of partners' discourse features is critical since communication is reciprocal with each participant shaping the interaction." They argue that conversational discourse by Alzheimer's patients needs to be investigated in ecologically valid contexts in order to discover the comprehensive effects of Alzheimer's disease on communication.

Perhaps the most obvious signal that a speaker is attending to his or her conversational partner's needs is whether the language used is one thought to be understood by that partner. In their investigation of code-switching by four multilingual Alzheimer's patients, De Santi, Obler, Sabo-Abramson, and Goldberger (1990) report that while their subjects' code switching was almost always linguistically correct, two of their patients no longer maintained the distinction between conversing with a bilingual and a monolingual, as evidenced by code-switching in both situations.

Another very basic issue in the discussion of participant relations is the relative symmetry of contributions made by the conversation's partners to the interaction. Causino, Obler, Knoefel, and Albert (forthcoming) report a tendency on the part of their ten late-stage Alzheimer's patients not to initiate communication, but to participate primarily in the role of responding to questions directed to them. This shift in the division of labor in discourse over the course of Alzheimer's disease is discussed in chapter 3 of the present study.

Within this component of Schiffrin's model, we can look not only at language adjustments made by Alzheimer's patients, but also at those made by healthy partners in interactions with such patients. As mentioned above, Sabat (1991) suggests that his adjustments of his own turn-taking behavior in conversations with one Alzheimer's patient allowed the patient time to find words and organize her thoughts. He argues that had he not adjusted his behavior, he most likely would have come away from the conversations with the impression that the patient was inarticulate, confused, and incoherent, rather than the thoughtful, sensitive, erudite, and witty person he consequently judged her to be. Sabat points out that we need to look at the healthy conversational partner's behavior as being capable of influencing the relative success of the patient's conversational interactions. This idea is elaborated in Hamilton (1991) and in chapters 3 and 4 of this study.

Ripich *et al.* (1991) also observed adjustments in the language used by the examiner in their study when talking with Alzheimer's patients. They found that not only did the patients produce shorter utterances in the interview than the healthy controls, but the interviewer also produced shorter utterances when talking with the patients than when talking with the healthy controls, creating "highly interactive patterns of exchange." In an earlier article, Ripich and Terrell (1988) had reported that the healthy examiner in their interview situation had used three times as many words and five times as many turns with Alzheimer's patients as with the healthy elderly individuals in the study.

In his investigation of topics in interactions between nursing staff and institutionalized patients, Nussbaum (1991) found that personal topics voiced by patients were typically not reciprocated by staff, and that the content of the conversations tended to be quite controlled by the staff. Nussbaum points to the influence of the institution on this situation, i.e., that there are often contradictory purposes in such staff–patient interactions. A nurse may be attempting to complete a task while a patient may be attempting to build a closer relationship by talk. In their examination of conversations between Alzheimer's patients and volunteers unknown to the patients, Smith and Ventis (1990) observed that although both parties contribute equally to topic development, the volunteers introduce new topics to a greater extent than do the patients.

Thus far, we have been considering only the participant framework of interactions between Alzheimer's patients and healthy interlocutors. Smith and Ventis (1990), however, found differences in the language used by Alzheimer's patients in conversations with other Alzheimer's patients from that used in conversations with healthy family members or unknown volunteers. They observed that the patients produced more minimal responses when listening to other patients, produced more statements of empathy and sympathy, and laughed twice as much. Although this work is only suggestive in nature, it opens the door to important future research on conversations between Alzheimer's patients. This is important because, as Smith and Ventis argue, the cognitive deficits so characteristic of Alzheimer's disease may actually not function as "deficits" when these patients interact with one another.

The preceding sections have provided us with information about language problems as observed in groups of Alzheimer's patients which may contribute to problems of local coherence in interactions with these patients. In the following sections I introduce the reader to the conversational partners and their conversations which comprise the data base for this study. It is my hope that the enjoyment Elsie and I exhibit in these talks will not be completely dissected away as analytical frameworks are presented and findings reported. I hope in upcoming chapters to be able to maintain some of the feeling expressed by Rust (1986: 140) who, as a nurses' aid, enjoyed talking with another elderly female Alzheimer's patient, Amy: "We sit and simply take up talking, wherever and whenever we are. Talking with Amy ... is a wonderful experience in which we are always in the present, and the present could be anything we choose to create between us."

Description of the interactions

Following Rosen's (1988) notion of "autobiography as resource," in this section I briefly discuss the process which led from my talks with Elsie to the analyses and, finally, to the writing of this book. I do this to bring into the open insights regarding my approach to research which might be masked in a more product-oriented discussion.

At the outset of my conversations with Elsie, I did not know what I would find. In 1981 when I got to know Elsie, very little was reported in the scholarly literature about language and Alzheimer's disease. I relied initially on Obler's (1981) insightful review of Irigaray's (1973) study of thirty-two Alzheimer's patients in France as well as on a volume on language, communication, and the elderly edited by Obler and Albert (1980b). But as a student of interactional sociolinguistics and discourse analysis, I was unable to find theoretical frameworks and methodologies in the literature which allowed me to capture what I sensed was potentially most significant about Elsie's communicative abilities and how they were interrelated with my own communicative behavior in our conversations.

In the face of the publication of increasingly numerous studies on language and Alzheimer's disease from a clinical or psycholinguistic perspective, I continued to ask myself what a sociolinguistic approach to this problem would look like and indeed, some times, whether it was possible. Insights from the first couple of years came primarily from Deborah Tannen, Deborah Schiffrin, and Roger Shuy. From Deborah Tannen I learned about work on face issues and politeness (e.g. Goffman 1967; Lakoff 1973, 1979; Brown and Levinson 1978 [1987]); Deborah Schiffrin introduced me to the concepts of "taking the role of the other" (Mead 1934) and "sociability" (Simmel 1961); Roger Shuy discussed with me the qualitative approach of ethnography, which enabled me to feel comfortable with allowing the conversational data themselves to lead me to my frameworks and working hypotheses.

This study, then, partly by design and partly by necessity, is a highly data-driven study. Sense-making difficulties and unusual moments in the conversations would pique my linguistic curiosity along the way and lead me to wonder about possible interrelationships in the data. But it was not until after the final conversation examined in this study that I began to use these observations and considerations to form the analytical tools and frameworks which would allow me to carry out quantitative analyses which seemed to be true to the data.

It should be clear from the preceding review of the literature on language and Alzheimer's disease that the longitudinal approach taken here can be potentially helpful in tracking the progression of the break-down of a patient's communicative abilities. In fact, it was noted in the discussion of the language correlates of the stages of Alzheimer's disease above that a somewhat artificial construct had to be built based on findings of a variety of synchronic studies of patients at various stages of the disease. To my knowledge, the present study is the first one to examine over real time the viability of the proposed sequence of communicative breakdown.

Regarding the appropriateness of the case study approach, a number of researchers have pointed out the difficulties inherent in group studies of Alzheimer's patients due to the variability in the nature of their communi-cative impairments (Sabat pers. comm.; Gardner 1974; Bayles 1985; Shuttleworth and Huber 1988). A quick glance at the standard deviations in many statistical tables accompanying reports of group studies indicates that quite significant individual differences are being averaged out. In their investigation of naming disorders in Alzheimer's disease, Shuttleworth and Huber (1988: 232) argue that "attempting to average patient scores may tend to confuse rather than to clarify." Despite these individual differences in test results, Sloan (1990b) reports that the relative strengths and weaknesses of Alzheimer's patients typically remain consistent from the initial diagnosis to the end-stages of the disease. Moody (1989: 228) calls for researchers to take a qualitative approach to help sort out this dilemma by looking "behind quantitative data to discern differences lost according to commonly used methods of data reduction. Where quantifi-cation offers the power of abstraction, qualitative data returns us to 'the things themselves' and to realities to elude conventional scales and instruments."

Of course, the flip side of this problem is the equally serious problem of reporting idiosyncratic findings in a case study (see Caramazza 1986; McCloskey and Caramazza 1988; Caramazza and Badecker 1989; Cara-mazza 1991 for a discussion of the viability of single-patient studies). Given the kinds of in-depth quantitative and qualitative investigations which must be carried out to get beyond a superficial characterization of disordered discourse, however, I would argue that a case study is a sensible way to begin identifying the interrelationships between a variety of language phenomena in discourse. These findings, then, can be used to develop principled research questions and methodologies for larger group studies. In their investigation of the discourse produced by a single Wernicke's aphasic, Ulatowksa, Allard, and Chapman (1990) argue the benefit of a case-study design to allow for a micro-analysis of the disordered discourse, which then can be followed by a group study to test the degree of generalization of the findings.

In this study, I am not claiming that the specific findings regarding Elsie's and my production of and responses to questions in our conversations over four years can be generalized to other specific interactions between other conversational partners at other times and places. What I am claiming is that an in-depth examination of language used by particular people in particular interactions will provide us with a heightened understanding of interactional influence on language as it relates to Alzheimer's disease, which may inform future large group studies. In this spirit, I hope to offer the reader (1) an alternative, complementary approach to language pathology based on natural, interactional principles, (2) a discussion of theoretical notions such as taking the role of the other, automaticity, and division of labor in discourse and the ways in which these manifest themselves in natural discourse, and (3) a critical discussion of some methodological issues relating to the elicitation and interactional analysis of discourse.

The observations and analyses reported in this study are based on fourteen naturally occurring conversations I had with one Alzheimer's patient, Elsie, which were tape-recorded in a 121-bed Washington, D.C.-area private health care center between November 1981 and March 1986.[9] In my role of participant-observer, I was carrying out what Kitwood (1988: 176) calls a personal research approach which is meant to supplement the technical approach normally taken in studies of Alzheimer's disease. Kitwood describes the researcher's role as follows:

The key to a personal approach is that it does not "stand outside," taking the position of a detached and unaffected observer. At its core, it works interpretively and empathetically, going far beyond the measurement of indices or the codification of behaviour. In all of this the researcher takes a personal risk . . . *It is on the ground of our own experience in relationship that we can gain some inkling of what is happening to another.* (my emphasis)

Because determinations of the extent to which one partner is interacting successfully *in a natural setting* rely on an insider's knowledge of what has been shared over time (see Blakar 1985 for discussion), I argue it is

9 I wish to thank Ms. Jill Bergen, former Coordinator of Volunteer Services, The Hermitage in Northern Virginia, for arranging permission for me to tape-record interactions in which I was involved at the health care center, and "Elsie," a wonderful woman whom I never saw only as an informant but came to love as a friend.

legitimate, if not imperative, for the analyst to take this role of participant-observer in an interactional study of communicative breakdown.

The conversational partners

At the time of the interactions, the patient, who will be called "Elsie," was
from 81 to 86 years old. My use of a first name for the patient throughout
this study is meant to reflect the situation as I knew it to be at the health
care center. There, staff members called some patients, including "Elsie,"
by their first names, whereas others were called by title and last name. As
an outsider to the institution at the beginning of my work there, I did not
question this differentiation and simply used the names in the way I heard
them being used around me. My use of the first name "Elsie" in this study
should not be understood as my condoning the frequent use of elderly
individuals' first names in nursing homes, which is often disconcerting to
those elderly individuals. It is a reflection of reality, and in no way is
meant to convey disrespect for the patient (see Wood and Ryan 1991 for a
discussion on forms of address and age and Caporeal 1981 for a discussion
of patients' perceptions of the "paralanguage of caregiving").[10]

Elsie had earned an advanced degree and had been professionally active
as a leader in the church until ten years before the beginning of this study.
She had an outgoing personality and was very friendly to residents,
volunteers, and staff alike. Elsie enjoyed taking part in social activities in the
health care center when her physical health allowed and was visibly pleased
when she saw people she recognized at these activities. According to the
Global Deterioration Scale (GDS) for Age-Associated Cognitive Decline
and Alzheimer's Disease (Reisberg, Ferris, de Leon, *et al.* 1982), Elsie was at
the stage of moderately severe cognitive decline (stage 5) at the onset of our
conversations in 1981 and had reached the stage of very severe cognitive
decline (stage 7) by 1986. GDS stage 5 corresponds to the clinical phase
"early dementia"; stage 7 corresponds to the clinical phase "late dementia."
At the beginning of the study, Elsie could walk and eat independent of
others' assistance; by 1985 she needed assistance to eat and drink. By March
1986, Elsie was bed-ridden and her verbal production consisted solely of the
responses *mmm, mhm, mm Hm, hmm?*, and *uhhuh*, although her systematic
use of these indicates a degree of comprehension on her part, especially of
personally important utterances (discussed in chapter 4).

---

[10] One of the reviewers of this manuscript indicated displeasure with my use of first names for
   both conversational partners, as it is in the reviewer's opinion "nevertheless demeaning,
   particularly reinforcing a stereotype of women." In keeping with the tone of our talks,
   however, I have decided to retain the first names for the interlocutors, and express regret
   for any offense it may cause.

At the time of my conversations with Elsie, I was between 26 and 31 years old and was no stranger to working with elderly individuals. During my years in high school and college I was a member of volunteer organizations that visited residents, including those with dementia, in area nursing homes. This previous experience interacting with institutionalized elderly individuals is important, I believe, in that it contributed to my perception that talking "just to talk" is a worthwhile activity to engage in with nursing-home residents in spite of the sometimes severe sense-making difficulties which accompanied these talks. My volunteer work at Elsie's health care center involved co-leading a weekly armchair exercise class and a baking class, assisting with afternoon parties, reading to blind residents, speaking with a woman who had lost her English abilities and could speak only her first language, German, and simply making myself available to "visit" with residents. Regarding the issue of names discussed above, I was known by my first name to the staff members, residents, and other volunteers at the center.

The conversations

The data base for the present study is composed of fourteen conversations of varying lengths and types which occurred in the course of my interactions at the health care center. The total amount of transcribed conversation is 4 hours and 24 minutes. The amount of variation in the length of the conversations, as well as where and when the conversations took place, is due to the fact that these segments are not planned interviews or timed conversational segments within a test battery, but naturally occurring conversations. These conversations were overwhelmingly driven by sociability, that is, we were "talking for talk's sake." This sociability is reflected in the fact that topics evolve dynamically throughout the conversations and, accordingly, that Elsie and I trade off being the "expert" as topics are initiated, maintained, and closed on subjects about which we know differing amounts.

In order to give the reader a sense of the conversations from which all of my examples in this study come, I will very briefly characterize each one.

1. November 13, 1981 (2 minutes): In this segment Elsie is on her way back to the second floor following a baking class on the ground floor. During the wait for the elevator with other residents and staff members and the elevator trip itself, talk centers on where we are going. The interaction ends when Elsie reaches her floor and a staff member takes responsibility for her.

2. November 20, 1981 (4 minutes): At the start of this segment I come

upon Elsie in the hallway on her way to the exercise class. As we wait for the elevator and make the trip from the second to the fourth floor conversational topics include food and a party to be held that afternoon. After we reach the fourth floor and are walking to the class, Elsie says that her leg hurts her. Upon seeing some nurses with food, she returns to the topic of eating. When we arrive at the exercise class, I tell the staff member there about Elsie's leg. Meanwhile, Elsie finds a seat and greets the other participants. I then pass out the equipment and the class begins.

3. November 20, 1981 (6 minutes): This segment follows Elsie on the way back to the second floor from the exercise class. On the way to the elevator, Elsie greets other residents and, in passing by the nurses' station, sees nurses eating lunch. Elsie makes a strong case for wanting to stop and talk with them (and to get something to eat). We tell her that lunch is waiting for her on her floor and succeed in getting her to the elevator. After arriving on the second floor, a staff member mentions a party to be held at 2 o'clock that afternoon. This remark sets off a confusing exchange due to Elsie's mistaking the "2" on the wall signifying second floor for the time of the party, 2 o'clock.

4. November 25, 1981 (8 minutes): This segment traces Elsie's route from the exercise class on the fourth floor to her lunch on the second floor. On her way to the elevator, Elsie talks about having a good time at class. In the elevator Elsie talks to a male resident. We take the elevator to the fifth floor where we let some people out. Elsie makes it known that she needs to go down to the second floor. Upon arrival at her floor, I take Elsie to her table to eat lunch.

5. November 27, 1981 (8 minutes): During an initial 1-minute segment, Elsie declines my offer to take her to the exercise class, because she is sorting out her purse. I tell her I will go to other floors first and return for her in the hopes she will be ready then. Then, in a 7-minute segment following the exercise class which she ended up attending, Elsie helps me to get residents in wheelchairs to the elevator, stopping to tell one man she is praying for him to get better. After reaching the second floor, Elsie goes with a staff member to eat lunch.

6. March 5, 1982 (41 minutes): Unlike the earlier conversations which have taken place in hallways and elevators as we moved between class and home, the first 30 minutes of this conversation take place next to a window in the lounge. There Elsie and I talk about a variety of things: the weather, Elsie's necklace, a new magazine, people and buildings outside the window, Elsie's son and husband, my home, and Elsie's travels. During the conversation, she cleans her eyeglasses and greets two residents who walk by. Because Elsie is cold in the lounge, we move to her room around the corner and continue talking for another 11 minutes.

During this part of the conversation we talk about the flags outside, photographs and porcelain figurines on her table, and letters from friends.

7. May 18, 1982 (8 minutes): During this conversation in the second-floor lounge, Elsie and I look at objects Elsie is carrying around in her tote bag, and talk about a new male orderly and an upcoming ice cream party.

8. May 20, 1982 (16 minutes): During this conversation in the lounge before our exercise class, we talk about my home and objects (a napkin, a paper cup, a hairbrush, and a drinking straw) which Elsie has with her. We look at Elsie's scrapbook from which she tries to read a letter. A staff member comes to manicure the fingernails of residents sitting in the lounge.

9. September 5, 1982 (31 minutes): This conversation in Elsie's room is framed by talk in the hallway walking to and from her room. Once in her room, we talk about a silk-flower arrangement, Elsie's scrapbook, the paintings on her wall, church bulletins and calendars of center events which she has collected, and photographs, greeting cards, and postcards on her chest of drawers. After I accompany Elsie back to the lounge where she is looking forward to eating, she introduces me to a friend of hers who is also a resident in the center.

10. October 2, 1982 (24 minutes): This segment begins when I come upon Elsie reading a book aloud in the lounge. After greeting me and talking a bit, Elsie tells me "I've been writing my letters ... so as to show what we can do" and continues to read aloud pages 12 to 14 which completes the first chapter of the book. Interspersed among her attempts to read are numerous instances of metacommunicative comments regarding pronunciation, difficulty of words, and punctuation markings.

11. March 17, 1984 (38 minutes): During this conversation in the lounge, Elsie and I are looking at and commenting on items in Elsie's mail order catalogue, including tools, pumps, chairs, windows, lamps, raincoats, sweaters, hammocks, and boat horns. At the end of the segment, residents begin to gather for dinner and the food arrives.

12. July 4, 1985 (29 minutes): During this segment, Elsie is in her room in bed and I am standing next to the bed. As she has a cold, I bring her tissues and help her to clean her nose. We look at old family photographs and magazines, and talk about the weather and the Fourth of July fireworks downtown. Elsie seems to want to get rid of the side railing on her bed.

13. July 12, 1985 (26 minutes): During this segment in her room, Elsie is in bed. I help her to drink water out of a glass, and we talk about the weather, old family photographs, meals at the center, and what day it is.

14. March 18, 1986 (23 minutes): During this segment, Elsie is in her room in bed and I am standing at her side. I get her tissues for her nose several times throughout my visit. We look at old photographs, magazines, and the book she was reading in the October 2, 1982 segment, and talk about Elsie's meals.

Preview of upcoming chapters

Chapter 2 draws a profile of Elsie's communicative abilities and difficulties as observed in the fourteen conversations and relates these to frameworks of taking the role of the other and automaticity in language. Against the backdrop of this communicative profile, then, chapter 3 compares questions produced by Elsie and me in five selected conversations over four years. Findings are discussed within a framework of division of labor in discourse. From this perspective, Elsie's decreasing share of the discourse work necessitates reassessment on my part of those abilities, resulting in a suitable amount of compensation in order to buoy up her competence level in those interactions. Chapter 4 then tracks Elsie's responses to my questions of her over time, pointing to qualitative changes in the appropriateness of her responses as well as to the importance of my accommodation to her decreasing communicative abilities. An examination of my responses to Elsie's questions according to the same appropriateness criteria results in the development of an interactional model of response strategies, in which a speaker's selection of such a strategy is determined by her relative focus on the interactional goals of coherence, positive face maintenance, and negative face maintenance. Chapter 5 brings this study to a close with a discussion of its implications for clinical applications, research methodology, and linguistic theory.

Becker (1988) is cited (Tannen 1987a: 238) as saying that the problem with science is that "it does not touch the personal and particular." This study of conversations with one Alzheimer's patient is offered as a "personal and particular" study in human-centered linguistics, one in which linguistic disability is seen not as an isolated phenomenon but as a human problem within multiple linguistic and social contexts.

2   Communicative profile of Elsie

In chapter 1 we saw that language problems of Alzheimer's disease patients seem to be not on the syntactic level, but on the discourse level. This chapter is meant to give the reader a general sense for the discourse-level abilities and difficulties of the Alzheimer's patient whose conversations are at the heart of this study. This communicative profile of Elsie should serve to contextualize the more specific analyses of questions and responses as presented in chapters 3 and 4.

This chapter begins with a discussion of the notions of taking the role of the other and automaticity of language. These notions then help us to understand Elsie's observed communicative abilities and difficulties as parts of a coherent whole rather than as unrelated occurrences. Against this comprehensive background, communicative phenomena which are problematic to the interactions are outlined, illustrated by typical examples from the fourteen conversations between November 1981 and March 1986.

To aid the reader who would like to relate specific examples to the larger interaction, reference is made following each example first to the number (in parentheses) which signifies the conversation's placement within the listing in chapter 1 followed by the date the conversation took place.

Taking the role of the other

Critical to an individual's success as a conversational partner is the ability to take the role of the other at every point in each given conversation. It is only by figuratively stepping into the mind of the addressee of our remarks that we are able to accomplish conversational coherence and maintain mutual face in interaction at the same time. Taking the role of the other is a crucial factor underlying the full range of linguistic and social decisions in interaction, such as whether to use a pronoun or a full noun phrase, when to take a turn-at-talk, and which speech acts, register, and conversational style to choose.

Mead (1934) speaks of the notion of taking the role of the other as being "basic to human social organization." He argues that only human beings possess the ability to predetermine how another person will react to their actions by evoking in themselves the same response the other person will have. Self-monitoring of one's own behavior continues, though, even in the absence of other human beings at a given time. In this case, it is not the *particular* other whose role is being taken but the *generalized* other. This generalized other is "the incorporation of the community within the individual" and is, in a sense, "the source of social conscience" (Cuzzort and King 1980: 109).

Sacks, Schegloff, and Jefferson (1978: 42–43) have applied the concept of taking the role of the other to participant behavior in *conversation*, whereas Mead's use of the notion of taking the role of the other applies to the full range of human behavior. Sacks and his colleagues use the term "recipient design" to describe what they call "perhaps the most general principle particularizing conversational interaction." In their analyses, they identify recipient design as operating with regard to such conversational phenomena as word selection, topic selection, ordering of sequences, and options and obligations for starting and terminating conversations. Erickson (1986) further differentiates the notion of "recipient design" into two types: (1) retrospective recipient design, in which a speaker takes what the interlocutor just did or said into account in the design of the emerging discourse, and (2) prospective recipient design, in which a speaker takes into account what she projects the interlocutor's reaction to the utterance to be in the design of that utterance.

Figurski (1987) outlines a model of person-awareness which further differentiates the notion of taking the role of the other. In this model, Figurski identifies three main dimensions of awareness: (1) target (the self or the other); (2) perspective (egocentric or allocentric); and (3) content (experience or image). The egocentric perspective towards the self results then in the awareness of one's own experience, whereas the allocentric perspective towards the self results in the awareness of how one is viewed (image) by the other. Accordingly, the egocentric perspective towards the other results in the awareness of how one views the other (image), whereas the allocentric perspective towards the other results in the awareness of the other's experience.

In taking the role of the other in conversation, interlocutors operate with various types of assumptions – including what constitutes shared background knowledge, world knowledge, social expectations, common sense, and cultural, ethnic, age, and sex stereotypes. When these assumptions prove to be wrong, and knowledge assumed to be shared is *not* shared, expectations are *not* met, or stereotypes are *not* confirmed in the interaction, interlocutors may experience interactive difficulties. Recent work represented by Coupland, Giles, and Wiemann (1991) indicates that these difficulties may be more prevalent than had previously been thought. Because of what Reddy (as discussed in McTear and King 1991) calls "radical subjectivity," miscommunication can actually be expected to be the norm rather than the exception. Following Reddy, McTear and King argue that "each person's view of the world is unique and different from that of other people. Communication is possible because there is sufficient common ground, but miscommunication is inevitable because the perspectives of each person are not totally identical." Characteristics of the conversationalists, such as age, sex, ethnic group, and disability, as well as their relationship to each other, can be expected to influence the type(s) of discourse strategies used in response to these major or minor breakdowns in communication.

Misunderstandings between members of different ethnic groups (Gumperz 1982; Gumperz and Tannen 1979) often involve unintended inferences on the part of the listener caused by interpretations based on a different set of cultural knowledge. Because interlocutors are usually unaware of such misinferencing, the source of the interactional nonsuccess cannot be pinpointed, and therefore cannot be as effectively smoothed over as in cases involving like interlocutors. This situation often leads to confirmation of stereotypes and prejudices about members of these other ethnic groups. In contrast to interethnic interactions, like interlocutors are more frequently in a position of identifying the source of a misunderstanding in the interaction. Once the trouble source has been identified, the conversational partners have the option to repair the problem (see Schegloff, Jefferson, and Sacks 1977). This repair can be initiated by the listener, in the form of a request for clarification of what was just said, or by the speaker, either in anticipation of some potential problem (prospective recipient design) or in reaction to something which she just said which might result in misunderstanding (retrospective recipient design).

Smoothing over the bumps in interaction between an Alzheimer's disease patient and a "normal" interlocutor of the same ethnic group is different from either the interethnic or the "same type" situations described above. In this case, as in interethnic encounters, we frequently find that inferences are drawn by the listener which are not intended by the speaker, or, alternatively, that inferences which are intended by the speaker are *not* drawn by the listener. If the interlocutors are members of the same ethnic group and have the same native language, however, the expectation exists that they should be able to operate under the same rules. If they are, in addition, both of the same sex, age, and approximate socio-economic status, the one critical factor which separates them is Alzheimer's disease. Any consistent interactional difficulties would then most likely be attributed to this disease. If, however, age also differentiates the interlocutors, the danger exists that negative evaluations springing from interactional nonsuccess will be overextended to include healthy elderly individuals rather than just describing individuals with Alzheimer's disease. Thus, the frustration resulting from such interactional difficulties can lead "normal" individuals to construct or confirm a stereotype of the senile population or the elderly population as a whole, similar to the reinforcement of racial and ethnic stereotypes as discussed in Gumperz (1982).

On the part of the Alzheimer's patient, the interactional frustration may result in a negative evaluation of the "normal" conversational partner or a social group he or she represents. Additionally, to the extent that the patient is aware of his or her disability, the communicative breakdown may heighten his or her own feelings of incompetence, leading to a potentially serious breakdown of mutual face in the interaction. In this case, the Alzheimer's patient may attempt to offer an excuse, however feeble, for his or her behavior which does not live up to expectations, indicating that he or she can take the perspective of the other (in Figurski's terms, an allocentric perspective on the self, resulting in awareness of how one is being viewed by the other person). Alternatively, the "normal" interlocutor may present a ready-made account for the Alzheimer's patient to accept as an explanation of his or her own apparent "temporary lapse."

In their examination of accommodation and the healthy elderly, Coupland, Coupland, Giles, and Henwood (1988) discuss the phenomenon of underaccommodation to conversational needs as a strategy sometimes found in the discourse directed to young interlocutors by elderly individuals. Characteristics of this under accommodation include greater focus on self than on the addressee and lowly attuned discourse management. Evaluation of elderly individuals by these young recipients of under accommodation is generally negative. For example, young interlocutors found elderly interlocutors to be inconsiderate, unhelpful, passive, or egocentric. An important distinction must be made, however, between the occasional *intentional* underaccommodation in which the speaker really does wish to be unhelpful to his or her conversational partner and the *unintentional* underaccommodation which I argue characterizes much of the discourse involving Alzheimer's patients. It is not the case that the patient does not *wish* to take the role of the other, it is that he or she *cannot* take the role of the other to the extent that "normal" interlocutors can. Unfortunately, this critical difference between ill-intent and disability on the part of the speaker is not always perceived by recipients of this underaccommodation, leading to undeserved negative evaluations of the patient's behavior.

With specific reference to Elsie's communicative abilities and difficulties as illustrated below, probably the most obvious manifestation of Elsie's difficulty in taking the role of the other in conversation is her misuse of the information system. That is, information which is *not* known to her conversational partner is presented by Elsie as given information, or information which *is* known to her conversational partner is presented as new information. Elsie's difficulty in using pronouns falls into this category as does her occasional introduction of utterances "out of the blue" into the discourse. Problems on the lexical level include Elsie's use of neologisms, her "reassignment" of the meaning of common words, and her overuse of "empty" words. On the topical level, topic shifts perceived as inappropriate by the conversational partner may indicate Elsie's underlying difficulty in determining what her interlocutor will view as an appropriate change in topic. As Elsie's ability to take the role of the other deteriorates over time, her own needs and wishes continue to play an important role in the interactions. Elsie's discourse abilities when dealing with personally important topics appear to be more flexible and sophisticated than when dealing with more banal ones. Additionally, Elsie's attempts to get the attention of her conversational partner and to indicate to her conversational partner that she did not hear her utterance further indicate her abilities to see that her own needs are met. Elsie's problems in interpreting indirectness used by the "normal" interlocutor can also be framed within the discussion of taking the role of the other. If Elsie has difficulty taking the perspective of her conversational partner, she may not be able to figure out his or her possible motivation(s) for using indirectness. Brown and Levinson (1987: 268) suggest that this is a general problem of indirect uses of language: "Decoding the communicative intent relies on the mutual availability of a reasonable and particular motive for being indirect."

Elsie's decreased ability to take the role of the other in conversation does not appear to be uniformly distributed across all facets of her language use. Following Halliday (1978), we observe that Elsie's abilities to take the role of the other on a more formal procedural dimension of interaction (what Halliday calls "mode") seem to remain intact longer than do her abilities to take the role of the other regarding the management of interpersonal positions, roles, and faces (what Halliday calls "tenor"), which, in turn, seem to remain intact longer than do her abilities to take the role of the other in terms of ideational content construction (what Halliday calls "field"). Evidence of breakdowns on the ideational content construction level, such as pronoun, lexical, and topic selection, exists in our very first conversations in fall 1981. Evidence of Elsie's successful use of accounts and positive politeness, which indicate that she can take the feelings of her conversational other into account, can be found through our September 1982 conversation. Evidence of Elsie's awareness of procedural demands of a discourse with regard to another's perspective, such as responding to questions and taking a turn-at-talk, can be found even in the very latest conversations in 1986.

Although the above discussion of problems in taking the role of the other has been limited to Elsie, and the upcoming discussion in chapter 4 of the use of discourse strategies to sustain the interaction focuses on my contributions, it is important to see that this distinction between disabled and normal is not hard and fast. Following Crystal's (1984) view of language handicap as an interactive phenomenon, I wish to point out that it is not only the Alzheimer's patient who has trouble taking the perspective of her conversational other. The distortion which exists because of the physiological problem of the Alzheimer's patient makes it very difficult, if not impossible, for the "normal" partner to take the perspective of her disabled conversational partner. As McTear and King (1991) argue, the miscommunication which exists in many clinical contexts derives from the discrepancies between the mental states of the interlocutors – the healthy participant as well as the patient – rather than from some problem in the linguistic channel arising only out of the communicative disability of the patient. "Normal" individuals and Alzheimer's patients sometimes employ somewhat different discourse strategies and draw on somewhat different resources in their attempts to deal with the uncertainty which accompanies their inability to take the role of the other; this fact, however, should not be mistaken for the assignment of complete inability on the part of the disabled individual and complete ability on the part of the "normal" conversational partner. Responsibility to make sense of what is going on, to attempt to accomplish conversational coherence, to save mutual face, and to sustain the interaction belongs to both interlocutors.

Automaticity

The concept of automaticity (Whitaker 1982a, 1982b) as discussed by Tannen (1987b) maintains that the more automatic a language feature or task has become over the experiences of a lifetime, the greater the chance that an individual will be able to use it appropriately. According to Bayles and Kaszniak (1987: 175), automatic processes are those which are "carried on without conscious monitoring." The phenomenon of automaticity is more easily recognized in language used by individuals with a disorder which affects various types of communication processes differentially than it is in unproblematic language produced by "normal" individuals. The fact that the more automatic phonological, morphological, and syntactic systems of a language are generally controlled much better by Alzheimer's patients than the more creative and higher-option semantic and pragmatic systems lends support to Whitaker's findings. Further, within the semantic and pragmatic systems, the more automatic processes, such as object naming and formulaic exchanges, respectively, are better preserved than more "effortful" processes, such as listing words within a category and drawing inferences, respectively.

In Kempler's (1984) study, the only task which was completed perfectly by all the Alzheimer's patients was the production of highly automatic sequences, such as days of the week and numbers. Sabat, Wiggs, and Pinizzotto (1984) report that one of their subjects, despite memory problems, could remember every word of prayers and hymns that she used to recite and sing in church. Another subject was able to play a number of familiar songs on the organ without sheet music. Fromm and Holland (1989) found that both mild and moderate Alzheimer's patients had less difficulty in communication using overlearned communicative behaviors such as greetings and accepting an apology than more cognitively taxing behaviors which involved the utilization of context. In their study of late-stage Alzheimer's patients, Causino, Obler, Knoefel, and Albert (forthcoming) found that these patients were usually able to interact appropriately when their responses were limited to giving "highly elliptical, overlearned responses to familiar questions" posed by the healthy conversational partner.

Cummings, Houlihan, and Hill (1986) show that, while Alzheimer's patients are able to carry out the relatively automatic activity of reading aloud until a very advanced stage of the disease, the more effortful part of reading, comprehending what one has read, deteriorates progressively along with the disease. My observations of Elsie reading aloud suggest that her ability to identify structural elements relevant to reading, such as chapter, page, paragraph, sentence, and clause remains intact even longer than her ability to read aloud fluently and accurately, which in turn remains intact longer than her ability to understand what she has read. In addition, my observations suggest that the level of Elsie's familiarity with the lexical items (relative automatic versus effortful decoding) strongly influences the level of accurate fluency of the reading. Clinical and everyday observations such as these led Bayles and Kaszniak (1987: 175) to state as a basic clinical principle that communication processes which are nonautomatic should be tested, since automatic processes carried on without conscious monitoring are those most likely to be maintained in dementia.

Besides the primarily automatic structural manipulations, such as turn-taking, which she is able to carry out in conversation, Elsie uses other types of language which seem to be more automatic than creative. These include language stored in long-term memory, such as culturally learned linguistic formulas (e.g. "Gee whiz!"), metacommunicative framing language (e.g., "I think"), and idiosyncratic ready-made language (e.g. professional jargon and terms of endearment), as well as language stored in short-term memory, such as immediate repetition of self and others, which can either be perceived as excessive (perseveration) or non-excessive.

In the rest of the chapter conversational evidence of Elsie's relative strengths and weaknesses in communication will be presented and discussed with reference to the notions of taking the role of the other and automaticity just outlined in an attempt to understand how these abilities are related to each other and how they change over time.

Conversational evidence of increasing problems in taking the role of the other

Following Figurski's insights into self-awareness and other-awareness discussed above, this section will provide conversational evidence of Elsie's increasing difficulty over time in taking an allocentric perspective of the other (other-experience awareness) and in taking an allocentric perspective on herself (self-image awareness). Evidence will then be provided which suggests that, as Elsie's ability to take the role of the other deteriorates over time, her own needs and wishes continue to play an important role in our interactions; that she, in Figurski's terms, is able to take an egocentric perspective on herself (self-experience awareness).

Other-experience awareness

Conversational evidence of Elsie's increasing problems over time with other-experience awareness comes from several communicative areas: (1) the responses to word-finding difficulty in interaction and the related problem of appropriate use of reference; (2) her comprehension (or lack thereof) of indirect speaker meanings in discourse; (3) her production of self-initiated repairs; (4) her production of compliments and expressions of appreciation; and (5) her explicit use of the personal pronoun *you* in various speech acts. We shall now address these areas in turn.

Word-finding difficulty As seen in chapter 1, word-finding difficulty is one of the earliest and most obvious manifestations of the communication breakdown which accompanies Alzheimer's disease. As would be expected, then, Elsie has a great deal of difficulty, throughout the fourteen conversations, in finding words. When she cannot think of a particular word, she sometimes coins a new word (neologism), talks around the word (circumlocution), uses an already existing word to mean something else (reassignment of meaning), uses a semantically related (but different) word, or makes use of a semantically "empty" word, such as "place" or "thing." The use of these different options seems to be systematic and, I argue, is related to her ability to take the role of the other, as discussed above.

Let us turn first to examples of each of these options as they occurred in our conversations.

Neologisms Example 1 shows Elsie's use of a neologism. Because neologisms are unconventional creations of the moment by the speaker, it is very difficult, if not impossible, for the listener to know what the referent of the neologism is. In some concrete cases, clues may be found in the environment of the interaction. In this example, Elsie and I are looking outside the window in the lounge on her floor of the health care center. The church I am referring to is on the other side of a circle drive and a parking lot in front of the center.[1]

Example 1

> HEIDI: Have you ever gone to that church over there? Across the
> street over there? There's a Methodist church.
> ELSIE: You mean these things in this little
> ringlim one here? Right there ⌈ where the
> HEIDI: ⌊ uh over

---

[1] Transcription conventions based on Tannen (1984):
A: ⌈ Brackets between lines to indicate overlapping speech
B: ⌊ Two people talking at the same time
Brackets on two lines ⌉
                       ⌋ indicate second utterance is latched onto first without perceptible
pause
: elongation of preceding sound (e.g. choo:se)
.. noticeable pause or break in rhythm
? indicates rising intonation
Upper-case letters indicate utterance-initial intonation
underlining indicates portions of the transcription under discussion in the text
(words in parentheses were not heard clearly)
( ) indicates that something was said, but it was not discernible
[words within brackets indicate non-verbal behavior]
In addition, where deemed relevant to the analysis or interpretation, the length of a pause is given to the nearest tenth of a second as measured by an electronic stop watch: (0.6) = pause of six-tenths of one second.

ELSIE: ⌐trees are?
HEIDI: └across from there.

((6) March 5, 1982)

The most likely referent for the neologism *ringlim* is the circle drive (or the grassy area enclosed by it) because of the similarity in meaning between *ring* and *circle*. Evidence from Elsie's subsequent utterance suggests that she was referring to the grassy area and not the drive around it, as the grassy area is *where the trees are*. My response to Elsie, which is simultaneous with her more specific reference to the trees, indicates that I understood *ringlim* to refer to some object or area between the center and the church because I directed her attention *across from* the *ringlim*. After several more attempts on my part to get Elsie to direct her gaze to the church building, and Elsie's continued requests for confirmation that she has understood, Elsie does seem to understand what I am talking about.

Circumlocutions Example 2 illustrates the use of a circumlocution by Elsie during a conversation she had with me about her son.

Example 2

ELSIE: So he's going to be back in a .. oh just
a few uh .. oh a couple of uh .. not a whole
day. ⌐
HEIDI: └uhhuh

((6) March 5, 1982)

In this example, Elsie is ultimately successful in narrowing down the options from within the set of lexical items which refer to a period of time (*minutes, hours, days, weeks, months*, etc.) to *hours* by finally saying *not a whole day*. This phrase immediately excludes the time periods larger than a day, such as *week* and *month*, and also makes the most probable referent *hour* because it is the next smaller unit of time.

Reassignment of meaning Elsie sometimes chooses a word from the English language and uses it to refer to an object to which it does not conventionally refer. Examples of this *reassignment of meaning* are sometimes one-of-a-kind occurrences in the conversations, such as is the case in example 3. Here Elsie and I are standing near her chest of drawers in her room looking at a variety of items displayed on the chest of drawers. Elsie points to a postcard and says the following:

Example 3

ELSIE: So and ⌐there's stocking.
HEIDI: └Is that from a friend of yours?

ELSIE: That's <u>stockings.</u> Yes.

HEIDI: Mhm.

ELSIE: "Dear Elsie" and it says "I hope you ..."

((9) September 5, 1982)

The fact that Elsie repeats the word *stocking*(s) following my overlapping question (*Is that from a friend of yours?*) before she answers *yes* provides evidence that Elsie's use of *stocking*(s) refers either to the postcard itself or to its sender (and not to a type of leg covering) and is not a random performance error for Elsie on this day. This usage of *stocking*(s) is, however, found nowhere else in our conversations.

There are, however, other examples of such reassignment of meaning which are not one-time occurrences. Examples 4 and 5 show Elsie using the word *dress* in two conversations six months apart to refer to paintings in two different locations. In example 4, Elsie and I are sitting in the lounge. I have just asked her whether she has any photographs from her travels abroad and she is having some problems with her answer. She then abruptly shifts her gaze to the wall across from us to some paintings apparently made by residents of the center. It is possible that my talk about pictures/photographs from other countries triggers Elsie's talk about these pictures on the wall.

Example 4

ELSIE: My <u>dress</u> .. my name is that one on the
     right ..⌐ the right one .. and this other
HEIDI: ∟ uhhuh
ELSIE: one is the one that has another one on
     it.
HEIDI: Uhhuh. Uhhuh. Yeah.

((6) March 5, 1982)

Elsie points to the paintings and says *My dress ... my name is that one on the right*, apparently calling her painting her *dress* and then correcting herself by using the word *name*. Although it does not result in the correct lexical item, this self-correction indicates Elsie's awareness that she had not chosen the correct word the first time.

In example 5, Elsie and I are talking in her room. Just prior to this segment, Elsie has been talking about her life at the center. She said that she liked the people and that she had a lot of interesting times there. Her next few utterances are unclear due to the large number of personal pronouns and "empty" words. She then apparently shifts the topic to two original oil paintings on the wall in her room, referring to them initially as *dresses*.

Example 5

ELSIE: And they have a uh those two those two
  dresses up above there ⌐
HEIDI: └ uhhuh. The pictures up there.
ELSIE: Picture. Yeah. And those are very good.
  One it was one of my uh relatives I
  think who (painted) that thing ⌐ and the
HEIDI: └ mmm
ELSIE: second one ⌐ too and
HEIDI: └ they're just beautiful
ELSIE: yeah and I think I think so too.

                                        ((9) September 5, 1982)

It is interesting to note that the same wrong lexical item (*dress*) is chosen
by Elsie in conversations six months apart from each other to refer to
different paintings. Despite this apparently long-lived "reassignment" of
the meaning of *dress*, the fact that Elsie is quick to pick up on the word
which I use to refer to the paintings (*pictures*) might mean that she is aware
that *dress* may not be the word she is looking for.

  Semantically related words   Another relatively common occurrence is the *substitution of semantically related words* for the words Elsie
actually should be using. Whereas no apparent semantic connection can
be found between *dress* and *painting* as in the segments above, in example
6 I have access to what Elsie really means (*reading* and *book*) by
comparing the words she is using (*writing* and *letters*) with her actions or
objects in the environment. Example 6 occurs a couple of minutes into our
conversation on October 2, 1982. I just found Elsie sitting in the lounge
with an open book in her hands. As I walk up to her, I notice that she is
reading page twelve of the novel aloud. She stops reading to chat about
my home and university. Then Elsie says the following:

Example 6

ELSIE: I've been writing my letters ⌐
HEIDI: └ You have
  been? ⌐
ELSIE: └ I mean uh (rea) these ⌐
HEIDI: └ uhhuh
ELSIE: so as to show what we can do. ⌐
HEIDI: └ Yeah.
  You been reading the book.

                                        ((10) October 2, 1982)

Here, Elsie chooses the semantic opposite (*writing*) of the intended word (*reading*). Her choice of *letters* for book is somewhat ambiguous: if the word *letters* refers to what is written on stationery and sent through the mail in an envelope, it can be seen as the substitution of a hyponym; on the other hand, if the word *letters* refers to the individual parts of the alphabet, then it can be seen as a part–whole relationship, since books are made up of individual letters.

"Empty" words   More often than using a neologism, a circumlocution, or a semantically related word, or reassigning the meaning of a word, Elsie uses what are called in the literature "empty" words when she is faced with a word-finding problem. These "empty" words include (*some*)*thing* or *kind* for inanimate objects, *somebody* or *one* for people, and *place* for locations. In example 7, Elsie and I are sitting in the lounge looking in Elsie's tote bag. Since I know Elsie enjoys looking through copies of the *National Geographic* magazine, I attempt to initiate that activity by asking her if she has a magazine with her.

> *Example 7*
>
> HEIDI: Do you have a magazine in here with . . pictures of other
>   countries?
>   (. . . . . this week?)
> ELSIE: of another country⌐ another country?
> HEIDI: ⌐ Uhhuh
> HEIDI: Yeah.
> ELSIE: Well, it's a different kind, but I
>   have. ⌐ So I have to wait later because
> HEIDI: ⌐ uhhuh
> ELSIE: we have to have work on <u>things that</u>
>   <u>go on</u> you know so it makes it better
>   much better. Yeah.

((7) May 18, 1982)

Her answer *Well, it's a different kind, but I have* indicates that she has a magazine with her, but it is not one with *pictures of other countries*. Elsie's use of the empty word *things* in her next utterance *So I have to wait later because we have to have work on things that go on* makes comprehension of the whole utterance nearly impossible. Apparently Elsie wants to wait with looking at the magazine because she has some work to do, but at exactly the point where we need specific information on what kind of work, she uses the phrase *things that go on*. Her use of "you know" following this phrase may suggest that Elsie realizes her inability to be explicit enough in this case and is trying to get me to take over a larger share of the discourse work.

As I mentioned above, Elsie's use of these different options in response to word-finding difficulty seems to be systematic. Following the conversations of fall 1982, Elsie no longer uses circumlocutions or semantically related words when she has problems finding a word. Instead, she continues to use neologisms, "empty" words, or reassigns the meaning of an unrelated word to take the "lost" word's place. In lieu of the intended word, the use of a circumlocution of a semantically related word indicates a greater other-orientation than does the use of a newly coined word, an inexplicit word, or a completely unrelated word. Clues as to the intended meaning are offered to the listener in the first two cases; in the latter three cases, the listener is offered at most an indication as to whether the speaker is referring to an inanimate object (*thing*), or a location (*place*), etc. That she stops providing a greater number of clues as to her intended meaning suggests that Elsie is no longer aware of the kinds of informational help she needs to offer her partner in order to maintain a successful conversation.

Elsie's difficulty in using reference appropriately may also be related to the word-finding difficulty just discussed. That is, if she cannot come up with the appropriate full noun phrase, she may use a pronoun instead, even though the pronoun does not provide enough information to the listener. These reference problems may, on the other hand, be traced to her problems in taking my perspective. In this interpretation, Elsie cannot realize that I do not have the referent for her pronouns in my bank of knowledge, and simply assumes that I will know what she knows. This would then be evidence of the egocentrism which has been discussed by Hutchinson and Jensen (1980) as a characteristic of Alzheimer's patients. According to this interpretation, then, Elsie's difficulties with the reference system would be part of an overall difficulty with the information system in communication. That is, Elsie presents information which is *not* known to her conversational partner as given information, or information which *is* known to her conversational partner as new information. Clearly the memory problems so prevalent in Alzheimer's disease may play a role in the patient's ability to assess what is new information for a given interlocutor. (This disruption of reference has been discussed at length in Ulatowska, Allard, and Chapman 1990 and has been speculatively linked to the problem in taking the needs of the listener into account in Ulatowska, Allard, Donnell, Bristow, Hayes, Flower, and North 1988, and Ripich and Terrell 1988.)

In example 8, I have just come upon Elsie reading aloud in the lounge on second floor. We exchange greetings and I ask her what she is reading about. She says she is *working on this*. Then she laughs and says *so that's was where she was (gonna go)* and immediately asks the following question.

Example 8

ELSIE: Where does she live? About the same?
    Where you folks do?
HEIDI: I don't know who ... who do you mean?
ELSIE: Oh.
HEIDI: I don't know who you mean.
ELSIE: Well, let's see. What street?

((10) October 2, 1982)

Since there is no apparent referent for *she* in the prior discourse or in the physical environment, I do not know who Elsie is talking about. My first question requesting clarification is met with a simple *Oh*. Elsie's utterance (*well, let's see*) following my restatement that I do not know who she means seems to indicate her awareness that a problem in understanding exists on my part. However, Elsie's subsequent reformulation of her question strongly suggests that she is unable to identify what the source of my problem is, namely, that I do not know who the referent for *she* is. Her question *What street?* is simply a further specification of her initial question, indicating that she is interested in the street name rather than the city name, for example. Given that Elsie has been reading when I arrive to talk to her, it is possible that the referent for *she* is to be found in the story. Her egocentrism would prevent her from realizing that, having just arrived, I could not possibly know what she knows about the story.

    Indirectness Elsie's problems in interpreting indirect speaker meaning as used by the "normal" interlocutor may also be framed within the discussion of taking the role of the other. If Elsie has difficulty taking the perspective of her conversational partner, she may not be able to figure out his or her possible motivation(s) for using indirectness. This difficulty in interpreting indirectness has also been documented in mild Alzheimer's patients: Bayles (1985) found a significant difference between mild Alzheimer's patients and normal subjects regarding ability to judge whether an utterance in a particular context was intended literally.

    Prior to example 9, I helped Elsie back to her room from the lounge where we were talking. We are now standing near her window in her room looking outside. Following a remark that she does not think it is going to rain, Elsie invites me to sit down. I need to go and visit other residents, however, and feel that I must refuse her offer to stay and talk.

Example 9

ELSIE: Please sit down.
HEIDI: Oh well, that's okay. I think I should probably go and see
       some more people but I wanted to come and talk with you
       this morning.
ELSIE: Oh <u>you mean,</u> wait a minute. <u>What what did you say?</u>
HEIDI: I just said that I should probably go and see a couple more
       people before exercise class starts.
ELSIE: Oh. for today⌐
HEIDI: ⌐ Uhhuh. For today. And
       then I'll be back for you when the
       class starts if you want to join us
       .. for exercise. ⌐
ELSIE: Oh <u>you mean</u>⌐ oh you oh I see
HEIDI: uhhuh
ELSIE: <u>you mean</u> then to look for us. <u>Is</u>
       <u>that what you meant?</u> ⌐
HEIDI: ⌐ I came to
       talk to you this morning ⌐
ELSIE: ⌐ mhm
HEIDI: because I think you're so interesting [laughs].
ELSIE: Well, you're glad that you can stay as long as you want to
       stay a while.⌐
HEIDI: ⌐ Okay. ⌐
ELSIE: ⌐ Yes. ⌐ (...)
HEIDI: ⌐ You've
ELSIE: ⌐You can sit right here.
HEIDI: ⌐ got such interesting things. Okay.
ELSIE: You sit right there.

((6) March 5, 1982)

Elsie has problems deciphering my very indirect refusal of her offer. My
reluctance to say *no* directly to her prompts her to ask me several times what
I mean, resulting, humorously enough, in a change in my plans. I end up
staying and talking with Elsie and visit the other residents later in the day.

While example 9 illustrates the problems Elsie has in understanding the
message underlying my indirect utterance, example 10 shows Elsie responding with a simple *yes* to a yes–no question which conventionally is
used to trigger a more elaborate response. In his discussion of responses to
yes–no questions, Yadugiri (1986) argues that a mere *yes* is inadequate in
pragmatic terms to such questions which are intended to check whether a

precondition holds for asking a relevant wh-question. In this example, Elsie appears to be responding to the *direct* reading, rather than the intended *indirect* reading, of the question. The fact that I follow up with a wh-question asking for more information indicates my expectation that the initial question would trigger a fuller response.

In example 10, I am trying to get Elsie to talk about her extensive travels and residence abroad.

Example 10

HEIDI: Did you ever live in someplace like India .. or uh Japan?
ELSIE: Oh yes. In other countries ⌐ of the
HEIDI: └ yeah
ELSIE: world ⌐ you mean?⌐
HEIDI: └ mhm └ mhm
ELSIE: Yes.
HEIDI: Which ones? Do you remember?
ELSIE: Oh I've been to quite a few.

((6) March 5, 1982)

In this example, however, Elsie merely answers *yes*. Her reformulation of my question about specific countries to a more general question about *other countries of the world* indicates that she has understood the question. That she has not inferred my *intent* that the yes–no question serve indirectly as a request for a more elaborate answer is indicated by her simple answer *yes*. In response to my follow-up question, *which ones?*, Elsie says *I've been to quite a few*. This response suggests that Elsie realizes a more complete answer is expected of her, but long-term memory problems or word-finding difficulties probably do not allow a more specific response.

Against the background of memory and word-finding difficulties, an alternative interpretation of this example is possible. Perhaps Elsie *does* understand initially that more specific information is being requested of her. Knowing her limitations in providing such an answer, however, she opts to answer the direct reading of the question. Only when she is pushed by the follow-up question does she have to lay bare the fact that she cannot provide such specific information.

Self-initiated repair In their discussion of organization of repair in conversation, Schegloff, Jefferson, and Sacks (1977) differentiate between self-initiated and other-initiated repair. Whereas the use of a self-initiated repair indicates an awareness on the part of the speaker that something that she has just said or is about to say needs to be adjusted to help the listener understand her correctly, the use of an other-initiated repair indicates an awareness on the part of the listener that her communicative needs are not being met by the current speaker. In that sense, then, Elsie's use of self-repair up through our conversations in July 1985 provides evidence that on some level she is continuing to take my communicative needs into account. Example 11 shows Elsie repairing her utterance by replacing the lexical item (*bree*) with the more readily understandable item *read*.

> *Example 11*
>
> HEIDI: What do you want?
> ELSIE: I have to (bree) read.
>
>   ((12) July 4, 1985)

The phenomenon of self-repair is also reported by Illes (1989) for Alzheimer's patients in the early and middle stages of the disease. Illes suggests that this repair work shows that these patients "were aware of their own verbal difficulties as well as the presence of the interlocutor."

Elsie's use of other-initiated repairs will be discussed in the section on self-experience awareness below.

Use of compliments and expressions of appreciation   Elsie's decreasing ability to take the perspective of her partner is additionally indicated by the fact that after spring 1984 she no longer gives compliments or expresses appreciation. These communicative tasks, which had been characteristic of her conversational contributions up until that time, are examples of what Brown and Levinson (1987: 62) term "positive politeness." This refers to the orientation of one's utterance toward making the conversational partner feel wanted and liked. Examples 12 and 13 illustrate Elsie's use of positive politeness in the center. Example 12 takes place in the elevator following the exercise class. Elsie is complimenting a fellow resident of the center on her dress.

> *Example 12*
>
> ELSIE: That's a very pretty dress.
> HEIDI: Isn't that?
> ELSIE: Isn't that pretty? Ye:s.
> HEIDI: It's lovely.
> ELSIE: You all have .. yours is pretty too.
> HEIDI: [laughing] Oh well, thank you.
> ELSIE: and you too. [laughing]
>
>   ((3) November 20, 1981)

After I support her linguistically in her compliment to the other resident, Elsie distributes compliments to all of us in the elevator, seeming to derive immense joy from making people feel good.

Even in later conversations when her utterances become more difficult to understand, Elsie's compliments are strikingly well-formed and easy to comprehend. Example 13 occurs while Elsie and I are looking at a mail-order catalogue in the lounge. At the beginning of this segment Elsie is still referring to objects represented in the catalogue.

Example 13

ELSIE: Now these are very (huse some of
    that day). Mhm.⌐
HEIDI: └ I think ⌐ I remember
ELSIE: └ Your hair
<u>is so beautiful.</u>⌐
HEIDI: └ Well, thank you.

((11) March 17, 1984)

During my time as a volunteer at the center, I observed time and time again that this ability to make others feel good was a crucial factor in Elsie's attracting conversational partners. Her use of positive politeness seemed in many cases to offset the uncomfortableness caused by the confusion and communicative breakdowns. By summer 1985, however, such compliments are made no longer, and expressing appreciation to the person who is responsible for a desired action is replaced by a favorable ego-centered evaluation of the situation (*oh that's good*).

    Explicit use of the pronoun "you" We can also examine Elsie's use of the personal pronoun "you" in reference to her conversational partner as evidence of her increasing difficulty in taking the role of the other and the concomitant increase in the reference to herself. During our conversations together, Elsie uses the pronoun *you* to accomplish the following interactional tasks: to request information about me, to check her understanding of what I said (*you mean . . .?*), to request repetition of what I said (*What did you say?*), and to request an action on my part. Elsie's increasing difficulty in taking the role of her other is indicated by the fact that after the spring 1984 conversation, Elsie drops her requests for information about me, but continues (1) to ask questions which are critical to Elsie's own understanding of the conversation (repetitions and confirmations of understanding) and (2) to request that I carry out actions which will benefit Elsie.

Self-image awareness

Conversational evidence of Elsie's increasing problems over time with self-image awareness comes from her use of accounts. Accounts are defined by Scott and Lyman (1968) as linguistic devices which are crucial to social order because they "verbally bridge the gap between action and expectation." Furthermore, an account is made by a social actor "to explain unanticipated or untoward behavior." It follows, then, from this definition that a person giving an account is aware (at some level) of the gap between his or her actions and social expectations, and that some of his or her behavior counts as "unanticipated" or "untoward."

Elsie offers accounts quite frequently when she cannot answer questions which she obviously thinks *should* be answerable. In all of her accounts in our conversations, as in the accounts reproduced here, Elsie says she *forgets, can't remember* or *gets mixed up* because either the quantity is too great (*too many, too much, several*) or it is *too long ago*. In example 14, Elsie and I are looking at some original oil paintings on the wall in her room.

Example 14

HEIDI: Now this picture says S: Steve B. Smith. Steve Smith.
ELSIE: Oh . . in this one? Here?
HEIDI: Yeah. Is that?
ELSIE: Oh: yes.
HEIDI: Who is that?
ELSIE: yes. I uh I'm
HEIDI: Is
ELSIE: ⌐trying to think of im. We've got
HEIDI: ⌐that?
ELSIE: so many of em ⌐(hhh) that I forgot.
HEIDI: your son or grandson or something
maybe? Mhm.

((9) September 5, 1982)

Here, Elsie gives an account for having forgotten who *Steve B. Smith* is. In saying *we've got so many of em*, she seems to be making reference to the large size of her extended family; i.e. that since she has so many relatives, she simply cannot remember them all. That Elsie offers any reason at all for her memory problems provides evidence that she is still aware of what is socially expected of her.

In example 15, I am telling Elsie that I work with the volunteer coordinator at the center, Jill Masters.

Example 15

HEIDI: Do you know Jill?
ELSIE: Jill.
HEIDI: Jill Masters? The person who runs all of the activities?
ELSIE: Well, I don't know. I've had so many names (that I it) sometimes they are hard to get uh pickly I mean quickly [laughs]
HEIDI: quickly [laughs]⌐
ELSIE: └ quickly ⌐
HEIDI: [laughing]   └ pickly quickly
ELSIE: Yeah.

((9) September 5, 1982)

In this example, Elsie offers an account as to why she does not seem to remember the woman who runs the center's activities in which Elsie participates regularly. Because Elsie has been exposed to *so many names, they are hard to get . . . quickly*. Again, the simple fact that Elsie offers an account at all indicates that she senses that she should know Jill.

It is interesting to note that I observed *no* account by Elsie after the September 1982 conversation. This absence may reflect the general progression of the disease and, therefore, the deterioration of Elsie's cognitive abilities. It is possible that she is no longer aware of the "gap" between her actions (abilities) and social expectations, which is the necessary motivation for account-giving in the first place, or that she is giving up trying to bridge that gap. This interpretation is supported by observations that at the same time Elsie stops giving accounts, she also stops making reference to her memory problems (*I forget*) and stops giving self-evaluative comments, such as *We're coming along alright* or *Oh, I can do an awful lot if I ( )*. Figurski (1987: 200), in his discussion of self-awareness and other-awareness, sees a direct link between the ability of an individual to take the perspective of another person and the ability of that same person to stand outside the situation and evaluate her own performance. "If we cannot consider the experience of the other, then we can never be objective toward ourselves."

On the other hand, the absence of account-giving may simply be an artifact of my question strategy *vis-à-vis* Elsie. Perhaps I am subconsciously "protecting" Elsie from potentially uncomfortable situations by screening my questions to her. Another example of this kind of "before-the-fact" face-saving technique is discussed in chapter 4, where I accommodate to Elsie's increasing difficulty in answering wh-questions by asking proportionately fewer of them and more yes–no questions over time. The cause of Elsie's lack of account-giving is probably a combination of these factors.

In her investigation of the responses of laypersons and clinicians to a videotaped interview between an Alzheimer's patient and an examiner, Campbell-Taylor (1984) found that observers considered the patient's account-giving to be "unusual" behavior after noting its frequency of employment. Indeed, not only the frequency of account-giving underlay the judgments of unusual behavior, but also the fact that many of these accounts were judged to be ineffective and/or insufficient excuses for the unexpected behavior.

Self-experience awareness

Conversational evidence for Elsie's continued ability to take an egocentric perspective towards herself (self-experience awareness) comes from her discourse abilities when dealing with personally important topics and her ability as a listener to request clarification or repetition of the speaker's utterance so that she can understand it better.

Personally important topics   Elsie seems to be able to deal with topics of personal importance to her in a more flexible and sophisticated way than she deals with more banal topics. To illustrate the relatively sophisticated level of Elsie's language *production* when she is dealing with a topic which is important to her, I have reproduced in example 16 Elsie's attempt to obtain food from some nurses. On the way to the elevators from exercise class, we pass by a lunch area behind the nurses' station. On this day the door to the hallway is open and Elsie can see the nurses eating. Elsie is on her way back to her floor to have lunch and is hungry.

Example 16

ELSIE: Hello. Just a second. I
    wanna make a ⌐( )
HEIDI: └Well you can just say
    hello from here.⌐
ELSIE: └I just want to speak to them and I'll
    come right away in just a minute.
NURSE: I'll see you, Mrs. Smith. Goodbye!
HEIDI: C'mon. They're .. they're waiting
    for us.⌐
NURSE: └ Bye. ⌐ They're waiting for
ELSIE: └ Yes. I wanna .. I want

NURSE: you, Mrs. Smith. You'd better go.

ELSIE: to stop though.

NURSE: They're gonna leave you. You don't want them leaving you.

ELSIE: But why can't I have one here?

NURSE: ⌜ Go downstairs. ⌝
HEIDI: ⌞ You'll be ⌟ You'll be eating

soon ... ⌜ okay?
NURSE: ⌞ (you) go downstairs.

ELSIE: Can I have one piece? ⌝
NURSE: ⌞ That's no good.

That wasn't any good. ⌜ That was stale.
ELSIE: ⌞ Well, it looks

good. All those up there are
beautiful things. ⌜ Why can't I have
NURSE: ⌞ Go. on. You're

holding her up. Why don't ⌜ you let
HEIDI: ⌞ C'mon.

NURSE: her help you downstairs and
they'll find ⌜ you some food.
NURSE 2: ⌞ Goodbye!

HEIDI: Yeah. ⌜ You'll be eating lunch as soon
ELSIE: ⌞ Oh. Oh all right.

HEIDI: as you get home. ⌝
ELSIE: ⌞ All right.

HEIDI: Okay?

ELSIE: All right. Thank you. ⌝
HEIDI: ⌞ Sure. ⌝
ELSIE: ⌞ Yeah.

((3) November 20, 1981)

In her first two utterances, Elsie makes it clear that she wants something (*I wanna ..*), but at the same time that her wish is not going to be a big imposition on me (*just a second, just a minute*). When these utterances do not get her what she wants, she states directly that she wants to stop there. When one of the nurses continues to advise Elsie that she should go with me before she gets left behind, Elsie finally gets to the real point; i.e., that she wants not only to stop to talk to the nurses, but to get some food there. She asks *Why can't I have one here* and then reformulates it to the less confrontational *Can I have one piece* when the first request yields nothing. Even the nurse's attempts to fool Elsie into thinking the food is no good do not have the desired effect. Elsie counters with *Well, they look good* and repeats her plea *Why can't I have*. Only the concerted effort of the nurse and me explaining to Elsie that she will have lunch as soon as she gets downstairs to her floor halts her insistent attempt to get some food.

The fact that Elsie can continuously redesign her utterances to fit the moment in the interaction (*unimposing* to *direct statement of wish* to *confrontational request* to *less confrontational request* to *counterargument* to *acceptance* of argument) to try to get what she wants shows a level of sophistication not evident in her dealings with less personally important topics.

Elsie's apparent ability to differentiate personally important topics from more banal topics in terms of language *comprehension* is illustrated in detail in chapter 4. There the systematicity of Elsie's meager linguistic production in our conversation of March 18, 1986 is examined as a key to her level of comprehension. With the exception of one token of *uhhuh*, all of Elsie's responses are of three types: *mhm* (62 tokens), *mm Hm* (9 tokens), and *mmm* (7 tokens). *Mhm* seems to serve primarily as an "all-purpose" repsonse for Elsie in this conversation, which is used to fulfill conditional relevance. *Mm Hm* (same as *mhm* but with greater emphasis on the second syllable), on the other hand, seems to be a *definite* affirmative response. In response to highly emotional utterances or situations, Elsie uses *Mmm*, as illustrated by example 17. In this segment, after helping Elsie drink some water, I tell her that I love her.

> *Example 17*
> HEIDI: I love you, Elsie.
> ELSIE: Mmm.
> HEIDI: You know that?
> ELSIE: Mhm.
> ((14) March 18, 1986)

In this example, Elsie responds to the emotional utterance with *mmm*, whereas she responds to the less emotional follow-up question with *mhm*. The fact that six of the seven occurrences of *mmm* are in response to situations such as seeing a photograph of her family, or positive politeness utterances such as being told she is loved or is a sweet lady strongly suggest that Elsie can comprehend personally important situations and utterances even at an advanced stage of Alzheimer's disease.

Other-initiated repair   Elsie uses other-initiated repairs in conversation which indicate that she is able to identify when she is having trouble understanding what her conversational partner is saying and to ask for clarification or repetition. Until our conversation in March 1984, she uses all six types of clarification requests as described by McTear (1985) based on Garvey (1977, 1979) relatively appropriately. During our conversations in 1985 and 1986, however, she issues only non-specific requests for repetition (e.g. *Huh?*, *Hmm?*). A non-specific request for repetition does not identify for the speaker what the problem source is (as would, for example, the specific request for repetition *You went where?*), but just indicates the utterance was not heard or understood in a global way (see Hamilton, forthcoming, for a more complete discussion of repair). Other studies of Alzheimer's patients seem to corroborate this finding that other-initiated repair is a communicative ability which changes with the progression of the disease. In an investigation of functional language skills, Fromm (1988) found that eighteen out of a group of twenty patients with *moderately severe* Alzheimer's disease requested clarification or indicated a lack of understanding when, in a role play, a doctor asked if the patient had been experiencing "Clasmapsia dostinnia." In an investigation of ten *late-stage* Alzheimer's patients, however, Causino, Obler, Knoefel, and Albert (forthcoming) report that none of their patients requested repairs of their conversational partners.

Conversational evidence of maintained ability to use relatively automatic language

Conversational evidence of Elsie's maintained ability to use relatively automatic language comes from observations of her ability to carry out procedural tasks in the interactions as well as of her use of ready-made language both from long-term and short-term memory.

Procedural tasks in conversation

Procedural tasks which Elsie is able to perform even in the later conversations are of three types: (1) attention-getting devices; (2) ability to indicate that the interlocutor's utterance was not heard; and (3) structural manipulations of the conversational machinery.

Attention-getting devices Even in the later conversations, Elsie still employs attention-getting techniques. These are usually in the form of repeating her term of address for the other person (e.g. *honey dear*) as in example 18.

Example 18

ELSIE: Now are you? (0.4) Can uh you put some of your (perries), dear? (0.8) Honey dear? (0.6) Lovin? (0.9) Honey dear. (0.8)

Honey dear. (1.2) (You well some of it was the re: uh rest.)
Yeah.

((11) March 17, 1984)

In this example, Elsie appears to be asking me to carry out an action (*Can uh
you put some of your (perries)?*) which I do not understand. This problem in
comprehension is due at least in part to Elsie's use of the neologism *perries*
and the absence of the preposition or prepositional phrase which the verb
put requires. Elsie gives me five opportunities to respond, each time uttering
a term of endearment and pausing between 0.6 and 1.2 seconds. The first
three terms of endearment are said with rising question intonation. The last
two are said with increasing volume, falling intonation and stress on the
first syllable of "honey." Her fifth and final attempt to get my attention by
use of a term of endearment is followed by the longest pause (1.2 seconds).
When I still do not respond, Elsie continues her turn.

Elsie's attempts to get my attention are not always this unsuccessful. In
example 19, she uses the more explicit attention-getter *listen* in combination with a term of endearment.

Example 19

ELSIE: They have they're have to get to get together, honey dear.
And they have to get. Listen, dear honey.
HEIDI: Yes, what?

((12) July 4, 1985)

In this case, despite the fact that I do not understand what Elsie is saying,
Elsie's use of *listen* in addition to the term of endearment is effective in
getting my attention.

Ability to indicate that the interlocutor's utterance was not heard
This ability, which was discussed above as a "non-specific request for
repetition" in the section on other-initiated repair, ensures that a condition basic to communication is fulfilled, namely, that what one says is
heard by the other. Examples 20 and 21 taken from the last two
conversations between Elsie and me provide evidence that Elsie can still
indicate that she did not hear her conversational partner even at advanced
stages of the disease. In example 20, I am offering Elsie a drink of water
before I leave for the day.

Example 20

HEIDI: This is some water .. water .. to drink.
ELSIE: (.. some of these things) I think I think see ( ) [clears
throat]

HEIDI: Would you like a little more?
ELSIE: <u>What did you say, honey?</u>
HEIDI: Would you like some more water? Would you like to drink some more?

((13) July 12, 1985)

Elsie's question to me (*What did you say?*) is strikingly well formed in comparison with her surrounding utterances in this conversation. Judging from my subsequent utterances, I understand Elsie's question as a request not only for repetition but for reformulation of my question. I design the following question to be more specific by adding first the noun *water* and then the verb *drink*. I also give the reformulations a positive orientation through the use of the assertive form *some* rather than the non-assertive form *any*.

In our March 1986 conversation, Elsie's only questions are in the form of *hmm?* All three tokens are spoken in response to yes–no questions including direct reference to Elsie, as illustrated by example 21.

Example 21

HEIDI: Do you remember me?
ELSIE: <u>Hmm?</u>
HEIDI: Do you remember me?
ELSIE: [smiles]
HEIDI: Yeah?
ELSIE: Mhm.

((14) March 18, 1986)

All three instances of *hmm?* in this conversation, like example 20, result in exact repetition of my question, after which Elsie responds affirmatively. As mentioned above, this non-specific type of clarification request is the only one of the six types of clarification requests discussed by McTear (1985) and Garvey (1977, 1979) which is used by Elsie during the conversations of 1985 and 1986.

Structural manipulations   One of the striking features of Elsie's discourse is her excellent ability to deal with the mechanical parts of conversation. Examples 22–24 illustrate Elsie carrying out structural operations much more intricate than mere turn-taking. In example 22, which takes place in her room, Elsie repeats the portion of her utterance (*a lotta*) which was overlapped by mine, showing her awareness that I might not have heard what she said due to the overlap.

Example 22

HEIDI: How about these flowers?
ELSIE: Oh yes. ⌐ There's a lotta
HEIDI: ⌊ Aren't the flowers pretty?
ELSIE: a lot of things. Uhhuh.

((9) September 5, 1982)

In example 23, Elsie continues on the topic of flowers while I introduce a new activity of looking at old photographs. This example shows Elsie not only repeating a portion of her utterance which was overlapped by my question (that she *fixed up* the flowers), but also answering my question (that the people in the photograph are she and her husband) after her repetition.

Example 23

HEIDI: Those are more flowers. ⌐
ELSIE: ⌊ Yes. Uhhuh.
    Aren't they darling? ⌐
HEIDI: ⌊ Yes. ⌐ Well what
ELSIE: ⌊ So we.
HEIDI: ⌐ is this? ⌐
ELSIE: ⌊ So we ⌋ fixed em up. We fixed em
    up. Well there I am. and my ⌐ my
HEIDI: ⌊ uhhuh
ELSIE: uh husband.

((9) September 5, 1982)

This indicates that Elsie is not only able to realize that she has to repeat what was overlapped to ensure my hearing it, but also can *simultaneously* attend to *my* overlapped utterance and provide a response to it.

In example 24, Elsie answers my question about going to exercise class issued in lines 1–2, but not until line 12. In between my question and her answer to it, Elsie asks three related questions, two regarding the time of the class (lines 3 and 5) and one regarding what the class is (line 7).

Example 24

1. HEIDI: Hi. Would you like to go to exercise
2.   today?
3. ELSIE: What time? ⌐ When?
4. HEIDI: ⌊ Right right now.
5. ELSIE: When?

6. HEIDI: Right now.
7. ELSIE: And what is that doing?
8. HEIDI: uh . . Well, you know that stuff we do
9.   all the time with the uh with the
10.   little cymbals that we have and we
11.   have a good time with music.
12. ELSIE: Well, I don't know yet.

((5) November 27, 1982)

Given her short-term memory problems, that fact that Elsie can still ask and receive answers to three related questions before giving me an answer to my question is quite amazing and is evidence, I believe, for the hypothesis that structural manipulations in conversation remain intact longer than content-level manipulations.

Ready-made language

Elsie seems able to use ready-made language in the design of her discourse. The term "ready-made language" refers to the prefabricated pieces of language discussed by Bolinger (1961: 381) which speakers do not actively create when they talk, but rather "reach for" from an ever-growing inventory of talk they have used or heard before. Following Tannen's (1987a) notion that prepatterned language can be understood to be on a continuum of relative fixity (in the sense of long-lived) versus ephemerality over time, I discuss Elsie's use of ready-made language according to whether it is relatively long-lived or ephemeral.

Long-lived Examples of relatively long-lived ready-made language used by Elsie are culturally shared linguistic formulas, metacommunicative framing language, and, somewhat less fixed, but still long-lived, her own idiosyncratic ready-made language.

Linguistic formulas Linguistic formulas, as illustrated by examples 25–27, are part of generally shared cultural knowledge. In example 25, Elsie expresses her desire to have me come to visit her again with the formula *I should say so.*

Example 25

HEIDI: Would you like me to come next week to see you?
ELSIE: Sure. ⌐ Sure.
HEIDI: ⌐ Good. Good. I'll do that.
ELSIE: I should say so.

((13) July 12, 1985)

In example 26, Elsie is standing in front of the elevator following the exercise class. She seems to be somewhat confused as to whether she goes down or up on the elevator to her home floor. After I give her the answer, she uses the formula *Whatever you say* to indicate that she trusts me to tell her where she needs to go.

> *Example 26*
>
> ELSIE: Don't we go down? ⌐ Huh? Do we go
> HEIDI: ⌐ Here. You go
> ELSIE: ⌐down or up?⌐
> HEIDI: ⌐ down.   ⌐You go down, Elsie.
> ELSIE: <u>Whatever you say.</u>

((4) November 25, 1981)

Just prior to example 27, Elsie and I had heard the quick tongue of an auctioneer on the television set which was on in the lounge.

> *Example 27*
>
> ELSIE: Oh, <u>for goodness sake. My my.</u>

((7) May 18, 1982)

Elsie apparently found his vocal techniques worthy of comment and used the formulas *for goodness sake* and *my my* to do so.

Metacommunicative framing language   Metacommunicative framing language stands outside the actual content of the discourse and comments on the speaker's relationship to the content, i.e., whether she understands it (*I don't understand, I see*), agrees with it to a certain degree (*That's right, I think, I guess, I suppose*), disagrees with it (*I doubt*), does not know (*I don't know*), does not remember it (*I don't remember, I forget, I've forgotten, I forgot*), or wants to have a moment to reflect on it (*Wait a minute, Let's see, Lemme see*).

Since there are few stances one can take *vis-à-vis* a chunk of discourse relative to the possibilities regarding *content* of the discourse chunk, and these metacommunicative comments are "reusable" in a variety of situations (and have been used over the course of a lifetime), I understand metacommunicative framing language to be a type of "ready-made" language. Elsie's successful use of metalanguage corroborates the finding of a case study by Andresen (1986) of a severely aphasic patient whose most fluent and coherent language was used to say (metacommunicatively) that he could not say anything.

Idiosyncratic language   Whereas linguistic formulas form a pool of linguistic resources which are available to any speaker in the speech community, I understand idiosyncratic ready-made language to be more individual and to a certain extent a product of the speaker's life experiences.

Examples 28–30 illustrate this kind of individual automatic language which is specifically *related to the speaker's past experiences*. Elsie's utterances in these examples appear to derive from a time in her earlier church-related career and seem to be produced more automatically than the surrounding ones. They are more fluent and contain verbs and nouns not found in her less automatic passages. In example 28, Elsie passes an elderly man in a wheelchair on her way to the elevator following exercise class.

Example 28

ELSIE: I'm praying for you, dear honey, to help you better. Is that all right, dear honey? Honey? Yes. Lots of love to you, dear, to help you. Yeah. We've been good friends, haven't we? Haven't we, dear? And then I can go on. and uh. You can do it, honey. I'll pray for you.

((5) November 27, 1981)

Elsie begins and ends what she says to her fellow patient with the fact that she is praying for him to get better and will continue to do so. She expresses confidence that he can indeed get better. Although these instances all point to Elsie's earlier career in the ministry, it is her statement to herself *and then I can go on* which seems most to differentiate this chunk of discourse from one which could have been uttered by any other religious friend of the patient. It seems to shed light on an earlier time in Elsie's life when she conveyed concern, love, and confidence to whole groups of people in need of it. When Elsie thought her job was done with one person, she could move on to the next.

Example 29 occurs in the midst of talking about a church bulletin (referent for *thing* and *it*) which Elsie has in her hands.

Example 29

ELSIE: And we can put this thing. (fold) it. Pull it up (and) pull it down. If they were in a hurry so they wanted me to get em out. I can just say "Go ahead and I'll take you over at such and such a time."

((9) September 5, 1982)

This example contains a number of indications that Elsie is talking from a previous perspective and not about her present situation. First, the

concept of being *in a hurry* is basically foreign to residential life at the
nursing home. So, even though we do not know who the referents for *they*
are, we can be quite sure they are people outside the nursing home.
Second, the fact that *they* wanted Elsie to carry out some action indicates
their confidence that she indeed will be able to carry out that action. And
finally, Elsie indicates she is in charge of the situation by saying that *she*
will take *them* somewhere at *such and such a time.* This is in direct contrast
to her situation at the nursing home, where staff and volunteers have to
take charge of seeing that Elsie gets from place to place.

Example 30 occurs while Elsie is in the lounge waiting for her dinner to
come. She is sorting through some papers (referent for *this*).

Example 30

ELSIE: Now we'll start with this. I guess.
HEIDI: With this ⌐ one. Mhm
ELSIE: └ Yes. I guess. Yes, that does. But it may (samly)
calling can call more now, so. Maybe he's home. Cause
that was their base, you know, when we were getting star-
started. She can do what she wants to do, too.
HEIDI: Sure. ⌐ I   ⌐ I think we're all just
ELSIE: └ Yeah. ┘
HEIDI: waiting ⌐ for the food to come. ⌐
ELSIE: └ Yeah.   └ Yeah.

((11) March 17, 1984)

In this example, we are struck by the contrast of the fluency of the
underlined utterances with the disfluency of the utterance preceding those
(*But it may (samly) calling can call more now, so*). The use of the relatively
infrequent word *base* following Elsie's use of *home* in the previous
sentence conjures up the image of a home base for people (such as church
missionaries) who travel a great deal. To complete the interpretation
along this line, Elsie's phrase *when we were getting star-started* would then
likely refer to the beginnings of her career in the church. The fluency of
this passage, however, clearly does not contribute to sense-making in this
interaction, as evidenced by my response. I do not refer to anything Elsie
has just said about the past, but rather state what I perceive to be
happening at the present time (*I think we're all just waiting for the food to
come*). The source of my confusion seems to go beyond the fact that I have
no indication of the referents for *he* and *she*. It seems also to relate to the
fact that Elsie pulls me into the past with her through her use of *you know*;
I simply do not have enough detailed information on Elsie's background
to understand what she is suddenly saying with such self-assuredness.

In addition to this language from Elsie's past which seems to be incorporated relatively fluently and automatically into her ongoing discourse, I understand idiosyncratic ready-made language to include other building-blocks which Elsie uses in a marked way in her discourse. These include her frequent use of amount terms, the utterance *That's a good idea* and the term of endearment *dear honey*, as well as the marked use of opposites and the conditional mood. These will now be illustrated in turn.

The frequent use of *amount terms*, as illustrated by example 31, is very characteristic of Elsie's discourse and is, I would argue, part of her store of ready-made language. In this example Elsie is responding to my question to her whether she would like to move to another chair or would rather stay near the window where she has complained about the cold.

Example 31

ELSIE: Well, I think right now .. I just as soon
      do it <u>a little bit</u> cause it's gonna
      gonna (change) <u>some of it</u> cause the sunshine's coming in.
      and one was for (growin up) just <u>a little bit</u> ago (did
      <u>great big part</u>).

                                                   ((6) March 5, 1982)

Her frequent use of these amount terms, especially *a little bit*, contributes to the impression of Elsie as a tentative, hedging speaker. Although it is not possible here to determine definitively whether this interpretation is justified, their frequency does seem to suggest that they are simply ready-made building-blocks being used automatically to produce a greater amount of discourse with little additional effort.

Additionally, Elsie often uses the evaluative statement *That's a good idea* in places where a positive evaluation would be appropriate as a response but where reference to *a good idea* is odd if not completely inappropriate. The fact that *that's a good idea* seems to be interchangeable in Elsie's discourse with the simpler form *that's good* suggests that it, too, is a building-block to be used automatically by Elsie in constructing her discourse. Example 32 is one of many discussions Elsie and I had about where my home was located.

Example 32

ELSIE: And where did you say your home was?
HEIDI: It's uh just a couple blocks from here.
     I'm ⌐
ELSIE: └ Oh I see. Oh that's good.

HEIDI: I'm on Walter Road. ⌐
ELSIE: └ You can do that.
That's a good idea.

((6) March 5, 1982)

In this example, after positively evaluating with *Oh that's good* the fact that I only live a couple of blocks from the nursing home, Elsie produces the pragmatically odd evaluation *That's a good idea* of the fact that I live on Walter Road. The automatic usage of this phrase is indicated by an occurrence a couple of minutes earlier in the same conversation. There, following my statement that I live very close to the nursing home, Elsie's initial, automatic response was *Oh that's a good i:* which she broke off (an example of self-initiated repair) and replaced with the more appropriate *That's very good.*

The term of endearment, *dear honey*, and its less frequent variant, *honey dear*, seems to be best described as an automatically used building-block because of Elsie's frequent and nondiscriminating use of it. Elsie addresses male and female staff members, volunteers, as well as fellow patients with this form. In the interaction from which example 33 is drawn, Elsie is asking me to help her get up from her chair following the armchair exercise class.

Example 33

ELSIE: You have to help me up. ⌐ That's right, ⌐
HEIDI: └ oh   └ good.
ELSIE: dear honey.
HEIDI: Sure I can.
ELSIE: That's right, dear honey. Yes. That's right now.

((5) November 27, 1981)

Given the memory problems which accompany Alzheimer's disease, it is likely that Elsie has found such an address form to come in handy, since it enables her to talk directly and pleasantly to a wide variety of people without needing to (try to) remember their names. On another note, the three occurrences of *that's right* used by Elsie in this segment may signal a transitional stage between a normal amount of self-repetition and perseveration.

An additional characteristic of Elsie's discourse which can be understood as part of her idiosyncratic ready-made language is her use of opposites within an utterance. Once Elsie has chosen the first half of her statement, the second half in a sense follows "automatically," as it can be produced simply by negating what went before. In example 34, Elsie is cleaning her eyeglasses and makes the following comment with the presumed meaning that sometimes she is successful cleaning her glasses and sometimes she is not.

Example 34

> ELSIE: Sometimes they'll go alright and other times they won't be.

((6) March 5, 1982)

In this example we note that Elsie is successful at negating the adverb (*sometimes* vs. *other times*) as well as the auxiliary verb (*'ll* vs. *won't*), and continues to use the correct pronoun (*they*) and tense (future). Elsie's only problem is the mismatch between main verbs *go* and *be*, which would not even have been noticed if she had deleted the final verb following *won't*.

In example 35, while Elsie is tearing up a paper napkin and putting the pieces into a paper cup, she evaluates what she is doing in the following way:

Example 35

> ELSIE: So that'll do it okay. I guess it's right here.
> HEIDI: Put it in the cup?
> ELSIE: Well, sometimes it is and sometimes it isn't.
> HEIDI: Mhm.

((8) May 20, 1982)

The perfect form of this fluently uttered statement, in which the adverb, pronoun, verb, and tense in the first half all match their counterparts in the second half, contrasts starkly with its pragmatically inappropriate usage at this point in our conversation.

Example 36 is a continuation of example 29 which illustrates Elsie's automatic "professional" language. In example 36, Elsie apparently alternates talk about the church bulletin we are looking at (referent for *this* and *it*) with talk about her hypothetical response to some other people unknown to me.

Example 36

> ELSIE: We can put this thing. (fold) it. Pull it up (and) pull it down. If they were in a hurry so they wanted me to get em out. I can just say "Go ahead and I'll take you over at such and such a time"

HEIDI: mhm ⌐
ELSIE: ⌐ and I'll put <u>it</u> in and see how
    it goes. ⌐
HEIDI: ⌐ mhm⌐
ELSIE: ⌐ And sometimes they forget and sometimes
    they don't.

((9) September 5, 1982)

After saying that she would try putting the bulletin in her bag, Elsie resumes talking about these people, stating *sometimes they forget and sometimes they don't*. As in earlier examples, this statement is syntactically well informed but hard to decipher.

Examples 37 and 38 illustrate Elsie's marked use of the conditional mood. In these cases, it is important to point out that it is *not* Elsie's formation of the conditional mood which is out-of-the-ordinary, rather it is how she inserts it into the ongoing discourse. This phenomenon may be related to what Obler (1981) interprets as uncertainty of response on the part of some Alzheimer's patients. As manifestations of this uncertainty in Irigaray's (1973) data, Obler cites patients questioning the information they give or offering more than one response to a question. Elsie's memory problems may underlie her uncertainty of response.

Example 37 comes from Elsie's and my first conversation following my return from summer vacation.

Example 37

HEIDI: Did uh have you been going to exercise class? or to cooking class?
ELSIE: Tonight you mean?
HEIDI: With Jill, this summer. ⌐ Did you go?
ELSIE: ⌐ Oh summer.
    Summer. There <u>would</u> be.⌐
HEIDI: ⌐ uhhuh.

((9) September 5, 1982)

To my direct question about whether Elsie went to the exercise or cooking classes during the summer, Elsie answers in the conditional mood, even though the expected answer is a straightforward *yes* or *no*. Here this may reflect an uncertainty of response caused by memory problems on Elsie's part.

Example 38 takes place a couple of minutes before the segment represented in example 10 above, which illustrates Elsie's difficulty in understanding indirectness in conversation. In this segment, I have just opened up the topic of Elsie's residence abroad.

Example 38

> HEIDI: You know I've heard that you you lived
> in . . different countries around the
> world. ⌐ Is that right? ⌐
> ELSIE: └ Oh   └ Oh you mean did
> living in different parts of the ⌐
> HEIDI: └ of
> the world ⌐
> ELSIE: └ of the world? ⌐
> HEIDI: └ Uhhuh.
> ELSIE: Oh yes. There <u>would</u> be quite a lot.

((6) March 5, 1982)

Elsie waits to respond to my initial question until she has put my question into her own words and received a confirmation from me that she has indeed understood my meaning. After I give her this confirmation, she says *Oh yes. There* would *be quite a lot.* As was the case in example 14, it appears that Elsie does understand my question, and is having problems with her response to it. Elsie may be experiencing a word-finding problem and cannot produce the names of the countries necessary to answer the question, or she may not be able to remember which countries she lived in. Elsie may be conveying this uncertainty by her use of the conditional mood.

The last two phenomena, the marked use of opposites and the marked use of the conditional mood, of syntactically well-formed utterances being inappropriately placed within the discourse is similar to Elsie's church-related talk and her use of *That's a good idea*, both of which were generally well formed but often ill-placed. This mismatch suggests the existence of a type of automatic trigger which releases these building-blocks within the ongoing conversation, resulting in occasional inappropriate placement which is only infrequently subject to conscious self-monitoring by Elsie.

Ephemeral Elsie's use of ephemeral ready-made language is illustrated by appropriate self- and other-repetition as well as perseveration, or inappropriate self-repetition.

Repetition Following Tannen's (1987a, 1987b) work on repetition and formulaicity, it is interesting to note that one of Elsie's residual abilities is repetition – both repetition of other's talk as "ready-made" to incorporate into her utterances (examples 39–41) as well as repetition of her own previous utterances (examples 42–44) to continue holding on to her turn-at-talk. It is important to note here that this kind of repetition of self seems to differ only in degree, not type, from the kind of excessive self-repetition (perserveration) described below.

Examples 39–41 illustrate Elsie's repetitions of portions of the contributions of her conversational partners. In example 39, Elsie is standing with a group of residents, a staff member, and me at the elevators following the exercise class on the fourth floor. Depending on the constellation of the group in the elevator, sometimes we go up to the fifth floor before going down and sometimes we go down first. Elsie is interested in finding out what our plans are on this day.

Example 39

ELSIE: Do we go down ⌐or up?
STAFF: └ We'll go up first. ⌐
ELSIE: └ Up first. Up first.

((3) November 20, 1981)

In example 40, Elsie and I are talking about where our exercise class takes place.

Example 40

HEIDI: It's on uh fourth floor. ⌐
ELSIE: └ Fourth floor. Oh I see.

((6) March 5, 1982)

In example 41, I am talking about where I live relative to the center in answer to Elsie's question.

Example 41

HEIDI: It's about two blocks down the ⌐ street
ELSIE: └ About
HEIDI: ⌐ here.
ELSIE: └ two blocks. Mhm. Oh. Well that's not so hard.

((8) May 20, 1982)

In each of these cases, Elsie's ability to repeat what her conversational partner says provides her with an important source of lexical items. This repetition enables Elsie to be released momentarily from her word-finding difficulties and offers the illusion that she is a "normal" interlocutor.

Examples 42–44 illustrate Elsie's self-repetition. In example 42, Elsie is talking to a male resident in a wheelchair.

Example 42

ELSIE: I'll push you now. Sure. Sure. I've
known you quite a long time. You're
a good man. You're a good man. Sure.

((4) November 25, 1981)

In example 43, Elsie and I are talking about a scrapbook which Elsie has with her in the lounge.

Example 43

HEIDI: This is a nice book.
ELSIE: Yes it is. Yeah. Yes it is.

((9) September 5, 1982)

In example 44, while cleaning her eyeglasses, Elsie says the following about a spot on a lens.

Example 44

ELSIE: Cause this one will come over and
this will come out and this will
come out. I think. Mhm.

((6) March 5, 1982)

This language is ready-made and ready for repetition after its initial creation by Elsie. In these cases of self-repetition, it seems as if Elsie produces a carbon copy of what she just said in order to be able to say twice as much with only an iota of additional effort.

Perseveration The phenomenon of perseveration, or inappropriate self-repetition, does not occur in any noticeably abnormal way until our March 1984 conversation, and, even then, it is not disturbingly frequent. Examples 45 and 46 illustrate the shape that this phenomenon takes when it occurs. Prior to example 45, Elsie and I were looking at a mail-order catalogue. She then changed the topic to one I could not follow due largely to the number of pronouns without referents in her utterances.

Example 45

ELSIE: So they got over and then we've had and then they get (two through them). She can have it after (sem .. semanuaway) ⌐

HEIDI: ⌐ mhm ⌐

ELSIE: ⌐ I'll tell her
anyway. I'll tell her. I'll tell her to say. I'll ask her. And then
I'll tell her. ⌐ (now this) ⌐

HEIDI: ⌐mhm   ⌐ Have you had any visitors lately?

((11) March 17, 1984)

Elsie's perseveration includes four occurrences of the phrase *I'll tell her*, as well as two other verbs from the same semantic class, *say* and *ask*. It appears that Elsie's perseveration prompts me to initiate a change in topic (*Have you had any visitors lately?*), in an attempt to give Elsie a fresh start in the conversation.

Much later in the same conversation, Elsie and I are trying to figure out what a particular item in the mail-order catalogue is.

Example 46

ELSIE: Is that the (twelve day)?
HEIDI: I don't know what that is.
ELSIE: Well ⌐ it's
HEIDI: ⌐ it says a "radar" ⌐
ELSIE: ⌐ it's still the
date. yeah. ⌐
HEIDI: ⌐ "radar reflector"
ELSIE: So we'll have to find out. Finds out. We'll have to find out. To try to find it, dear.

((11) March 17, 1984)

In this example, Elsie's perseveration consists of four utterances containing the verb *find*, two exact repetitions *We'll have to find out*, one *finds out*, and one *to try to find it*. The trigger for this occurrence of perseveration seems to be our unfamiliarity with an object in the mail-order catalogue. In this case, Elsie's impulse to want to find out the answer is appropriate; the form it takes in the conversation is not.

Whereas perseveration in the conversations prior to summer 1985, as illustrated above, had a "word-play" character, where verbs and prepositions were combined and recombined (*they total em up they total em*

up and set em out and get em out and then have em get on to get in), in
summer 1985 perseveration takes the form of repetition of a single word (*I
will have to. hold hold hold hold hold this [there]*). Shindler, Caplan, and
Hier (1984) suggest that perseveration is related to the patient's inability
to self-monitor speech. My data tend to argue against this interpretation,
as evidence of self-initiated self-repair is found at every stage in which
perseveration occurs.

In tracking Elsie's use of ready-made language over time, it appears that
the more idiosyncratic language is lost before the more culturally shared
linguistic formulas. The marked use of *that's a good idea*, the professional
language, the overuse of amount terms, and the use of opposites,
discussed above as being characteristic of Elsie's discourse, all appear for
the last time in the March 1984 conversation. The only one of Elsie's
"personal" ready-made language characteristics to occur in summer 1985
is the use of terms of endearment. On the other hand, more general ready-
made language features, such as metacommunicative comments and
linguistic formulas (*Gee whiz!, I should say so*) continue to occur in
summer 1985, as does the more ephemeral repetition of the conversational
partner and repetition of self in the form of perseveration. Since the
idiosyncratic ready-made language phenomena are arguably what make a
chunk of discourse "Elsie's talk" as opposed to someone else's, this
finding fits well with the frequently observed personality changes noted by
family members of Alzheimer's patients (see Bayles and Kaszniak 1987
and Campbell-Taylor 1984). It could well be that part of the reason the
patient is "not the person I used to know" is that she or he is not using the
language "I used to know."

Summary

This chapter was meant to introduce the reader to a broad range of Elsie's
language use as I observed it during our fourteen tape-recorded conversations over four-and-one-half years. I first discussed two general notions,
taking the role of the other and automaticity of language, which served
then as a framework within which we could understand the relatedness of
the constellation of phenomena in Elsie's communicative profile rather
than viewing them as a mixed bag of unrelated problems. I hope that the
discussion in this chapter with its numerous illustrations has not only
offered insights into Elsie's language use, but has also breathed some life
into the descriptions of the conversational partners and the individual
conversations presented in chapter 1. It should serve as a rich context for
the more specific analyses of questions and responses presented in
chapters 3 and 4.

3 Questions

Maintaining coherent interaction which is socially acceptable to both conversational partners against the backdrop of communicative problems as discussed in chapter 2 is not easy. Choices need to be made regarding how to deal with the nonsuccess. In an attempt to ward off or lessen the threat of a breakdown, the "normal" interlocutor can accommodate "before-the-fact" to the disabled partner's communicative abilities and difficulties, allowing the disabled interlocutor to function at a higher level than would otherwise be possible. This preventive strategy is only effective, of course, if the "normal" individual's perceptions of the disabled individual's abilities match actual ability, i.e., that they do not result in overaccommodation.

In this chapter, I examine 518 questions asked by Elsie and me in five selected conversations. Within a framework of division of labor in discourse, many of the relationships between Elsie's and my question production can be understood. When Elsie produces increasingly fewer questions, I produce more. When Elsie seems less able to respond linguistically to my questions, I produce more questions which can be answered by actions, not words. When Elsie seems less able to talk about distant people, objects, and events, I make increasing use of proximal reference. Further, the next chapter, which analyses response strategies, will provide evidence that Elsie's decreasing ability to respond appropriately to wh-questions is met by my increased numbers of yes–no questions to her rather than wh-questions. All of these measures are examples of ways in which one conversational partner can do an increasingly large amount of the discourse work in order to buoy up the interaction in face of evidence of the other's decreased ability to carry out a particular discourse task. However, my perceptions of the discourse work which I need to carry out in order to compensate for Elsie's decreasing abilities may be off-target. These misperceptions lead me, for example, to make greater reference to the present time and to concrete objects than Elsie actually does. We see then that, whereas accurate assessments of which discourse tasks can and cannot be accomplished by the conversational partner lead to increased interactional success, inaccurate assessments may create a situation in which that partner is not given the opportunity to show what she can do.

Why study question/response pairs?

Merritt (1976: 329) maintains that "judgments of coherence involve primarily the hearer's expectations of what is to follow. In examining a question-next utterance sequence, the coherence of that next utterance as a follower of the question is determined by the constraints that the question places on the hearer's expectations." It is this relationship between question/response pairs and coherence which was the primary factor influencing me to focus in this study on questions and the responses which follow them. As has been discussed earlier, the problems in conversations with Alzheimer's patients are most noticeable at the discourse level; utterances which appear normal as isolated sentences suddenly become "bizarre" and (at least somewhat) incoherent within the context of the larger discourse. If we wish to uncover the factors underlying this incoherence, we cannot focus on sentence-internal phenomena such as word-finding problems, but must instead concentrate on phenomena which cross sentence boundaries.

Further, the difficulty which the Alzheimer's patient has in taking the role of his or her conversational partner makes an examination of the patient's dialogic discourse much more interesting and relevant than his or her monologic discourse. Questions and their responses presented themselves as a frequently occurring as well as a relatively easy-to-identify dialogic discourse phenomenon in the conversations I studied.

In this endeavor, it should be noted that I am not trying to find "what might distinguish a sequence of sentences that formed a discourse from a random sequence of sentences" (Merritt 1976: 316) in the sense of a discrete property of "discourse-hood," but rather am trying to identify criteria which will assist in (more or less objectively) identifying why a chunk of discourse subjectively seems to be more or less coherent (discourse-like) than another. Ripich and Terrell (1988: 14) argue that "To say a speaker is incoherent is to say that we as listeners cannot understand or follow the conversation. In one sense the listener is making a statement about his own confusion. There is no clear understanding of where the listener's tolerance level for incoherence lies." In my examination of questions and their responses, I am attempting to find systematic linguistic evidence to back up my more subjective characterization of these conversations. The criteria will help us to trace Elsie's production of questions and responses over time.

Several properties of question/response pairs make them an excellent data base with which to carry out longitudinal analyses of communicative difficulties as manifested in natural interactions with an Alzheimer's patient.

Intersubjectivity: First of all, the mere fact of asking and answering a question indicates a willingness and ability to take the role of the other person engaged in the conversation, or at least acknowledges that the other person is present. If Elsie initiates a question or designs a response to my question, it indicates that she is aware to some extent of our differing stores of knowledge.

Conditional relevance: A question sets up the expectation that an answer will follow. In fact, Goody (1978: 23) says that "the most general thing we can say about a question is that it compels, requires, may even demand, a response." If the answer is not provided, "it can be seen to be officially absent" (Schegloff 1968). This structural phenomenon allows us to provide evidence for Elsie's differential abilities regarding structure and content, as she seems aware of the fact that questions deserve responses, although she is not always sure what the content of those responses should be.

Evidence of understanding: In providing an answer to a question, Coulthard (1977) maintains that the person to whom the question is directed "is forced to show whether he did or did not understand what went before." This phenomenon is central to any study which has misunderstandings and communicative nonsuccesses at its heart. Work on the necessary prevalence of misunderstanding in everyday interaction (see Coupland, Giles, and Wiemann 1991; Goffman 1981) cautions us, however, about thinking that we can determine whether an interlocutor has actually understood what has just been said. Goffman (1981: 45) argues that "a respondent cannot make evident that he has understood *the* meaning of a statement, because in a sense there isn't one. All he can do is to respond to what he can display as *a* meaning that will carry – although, of course, he may effectively sustain the impression (and himself believe) that his *a* is the *the*."

Face and indirectness: Questions and responses can both be direct and indirect. Moeschler (1986) states that the following pairings are possible: direct question and direct response, direct question and indirect response, indirect question and direct response, indirect question and indirect response. The questioner's and responder's option not to say directly what is meant allows us to examine possible face motivations for that indirectness as well as the degree of understandability of that indirectness.

Role of questions in diagnosis and assessment: It is important to examine question/response routines in natural conversations with an Alzheimer's patient, because the diagnosis/assessment of an Alzheimer's patient is based in part on the patient's responses to a tester's questions. Campbell-Taylor (1984) notes the importance of a patient's communicative ability to the diagnosis of Alzheimer's disease: "Having ruled out focal neurological disease, the physician makes a diagnostic decision based *on the answers given by the patient and the behavior observed during the interview*" (my emphasis). In the artificial speech situations created in these interviews, often the patient performs miserably. Either the patient provides grossly inappropriate responses or simply does not respond. Could it be that the artificial setting inhibits the Alzheimer's patient from performing to the degree to which she is able within a natural setting? Perhaps questions out of context simply do not make sense to the patient. Crystal (1984: 109) makes the point that "seeing a reason for a question is often part of the information needed in order to know how to answer." What we learn about a patient's ability to ask and respond to questions in a relaxed, natural setting may help us to create more fitting and differentiated diagnostic tasks. My point here is *not* that all of the difficulties Alzheimer's patients have in communicating are artifacts of an artificial assessment situation; the range of communicative difficulties Elsie has in natural conversations was made evident in chapter 2. My point, rather, is that some of a patient's communicative behavior characterized as inappropriate may be a direct result of interactional factors, either those related to the interactional setting or to the healthy interlocutor's behavior, or both.

Division of labor: Finally, depending on the perceived degree of appropriateness of the interlocutor's responses to one's own questions, one can alter his or her share of the discourse labor by asking more or fewer questions than the other, answering his or her own questions, or altering the type of question asked to demand less work from the other. It is a more detailed discussion of what is meant by division of labor in discourse to which we now turn.

Division of labor in discourse

Division of labor in discourse is a notion which operates on the assumption that communication is achieved through the interaction of speaker and listener. The speaker has encoding work to do and, in turn, the listener has decoding and interpretation work to do. Division of labor refers to the relative amounts of work which the conversational partners contribute to the greater goals of making sense of what is going on, attempting to accomplish conversational coherence, saving mutual face and sustaining the interaction. This discourse work can be in the form of structural/sequential work, such as taking or relinquishing a turn-at-talk, which keeps the conversational mechanism going; face work, such as saving the partner from embarrassment; and ideational content work, such as selecting a topic (speaker's work) or drawing an inference (listener's work) from an indirectly stated utterance. The listener may be asked to call on knowledge from shared experiences with the speaker or from generally known cultural and world knowledge in order to make sense of what the speaker is saying. Regarding work on the speaker's side, he or she needs to realize when pieces of information critical to the understanding of his or her linguistic contribution are not yet part of the listener's knowledge bank. Indeed, this is the source of some of the interactional trouble in conversations with Alzheimer's patients in roles as either speaker or listener – due to memory problems or a more general cognitive breakdown, this assumed shared knowledge may not be accessible to these patients.

There are at least two levels of motivation behind the division of labor in discourse – one relating to production and the other to comprehension of discourse. The speaker has an easier time in the production of discourse if the listener takes some of the "load" off the speaker, such as being able to infer or generalize from what the speaker has said. And the listener has an easier time in comprehending the discourse if the speaker takes over a larger share of discourse labor by keeping the listener's perspective in mind. In her discussion of "audience participation in sense making," Tannen (1984: 156–157) speaks of interpersonal benefits that can be won by sharing the discourse labor. In forcing the listener to work to understand indirectness, the speaker can "achieve the sense of rapport that comes from being understood without saying what one means." At the same time, the listener is moved through his or her interpersonal involvement to identify emotionally with the speaker's beliefs, rather than having to be convinced through a rational argument.

The motivations on the part of the listener and the speaker seem then to represent the extreme poles of a tension inherent in any given discourse – a speaker would have an easier time if he or she were able to ramble egocentrically, not planning his or her discourse with the listener's needs in mind, thereby forcing the listener to do an overly large part of the understanding work. On the other hand, the listener would have an easier time if the speaker were able to elaborate completely and fully each of his or her conversational contributions, but as Garfinkel (1972) and his students have shown us, this is an "impossible assignment." In reality, these extreme versions do not exist. Rather, conversation is an achievement of both speaker and listener. As Bakhtin has eloquently stated (cited in McDermott and Tylbor 1983): "Language . . . lies on the borderline between oneself and the other. The word in language is half someone else's."

What counts as a question? Sequence, form, and function

As straightforward as it may seem at first blush, it is no easy task to define the terms "question" and "response." In his review of two studies on questions, Moeschler (1986) points to the common problem of a circular definition by citing Stenström (1984: 24–25): a question is "an utterance that may elicit an R (response)"; a response is "an utterance elicited by Q (question)." Goffman (1981: 51) suggests that another problematic definition is that of Schegloff and Sacks (1973: 299), who maintain that "finding an utterance to be an answer" can only be done "by consulting its sequential placement, e.g., its placement after a question." Goffman asks how it is that an inappropriate answer could be recognized if absolutely *anything* in the slot following a question counts per definition as an answer. Merritt (1976) asks the logical question: if the utterance following a question is not an answer (if it is, for example, another question) does that mean the discourse is incoherent? Or does the second question count as an answer?

Moeschler (1986) also finds the "elicitation" and "sequential" criteria to be insufficient for differentiating questions from their responses. He maintains "Q imposes constraints on R (illocutionary and discursive) and thus gives indications about what is a possible appropriate R and a possible inappropriate R, whereas R indicates only that certain conditions are satisfied relative to Q" (Moeschler 1986: 240). This approach, unlike earlier described approaches, not only addresses the problem of determining which utterances count as questions and which as responses, but also the problem of differentiating between appropriate and inappropriate responses.

Stenström (1984: 58) carries this differentiation further, to the point of setting up a typology of responses to questions. This typology includes (1) appropriate responses which consist of answers (which give the information requested) and replies (which evade or disclaim); (2) delayed responses, such as requests for repetition and clarification; and (3) inappropriate responses, which include silence or change of topic.[1]

Up until now, the work we have been discussing has been more concerned with the location of the utterance defined as a "question" relative to utterances it elicits and/or constrains than about what actually fills that slot, i.e. the form the question takes. Goody (1978) discusses two

---

[1] This article did not come to my attention until months after I had drawn up and applied the response evaluation criteria used in this study.

different types of question which are commonly known in the literature as yes–no and wh-questions. She observes that questions which are answered only with *yes* or *no* are already complete propositions, which only need confirmation or denial, as opposed to wh-questions for which the answer provides the missing clause to the incomplete proposition. Yadugiri (1986), however, points out that from the viewpoint of pragmatics, a simple *yes* or *no* to a yes–no question may actually be inadequate, if, for example, a yes–no question is meant as an indirect wh-question (see page 52, example 10, for an illustration). Robinson and Rackstraw (1972), in calling these two classes "open questions" and "closed questions," refer to the status of the propositional content in each case. Stubbs (1983) observes that, while a question termed a "yes–no question" is defined by the response to it (*yes* or *no*), a question termed a "wh-question" is defined by a subset of words which occur at the beginning of the question (*where, when, who, whose, which, what*, and *how*). In order to emphasize the type of response elicited by *both* types of questions, and therefore to move beyond sentence-level concerns to discourse issues, Stubbs (1983) uses the term "x-question" rather than "wh-question." Within his discussion of yes–no questions, Stubbs makes the important point that, while such questions do not always receive the responses *yes* or *no*, whatever follows a yes–no question will be interpreted as meaning either *yes* or *no*. Quirk, Greenbaum, Leech, and Svartvik (1972) divide questions into three major classes according to the type of response they expect, adding to yes–no questions and wh-questions what they call "alternative questions." This type of question expects as a response one or more of the alternatives mentioned in the question, such as *Do you want to go to your room or stay here in the lounge?*

Besides discussing the sequential position a question takes or its form, it is possible to examine the function(s) it fulfills. Vital to any discussion of linguistic function is work on "speech acts" pioneered by Austin (1962) and Searle (1969, 1975). These language philosophers argued convincingly that, in talking, we not only talk, but perform (social) acts. For example, as I utter words to promise (or threaten or warn) that I will clean up the apartment (explicitly or not) I am carrying out the act of promising (or threatening or warning). Their related point that syntactic form and communicative function do not necessarily mesh is of critical importance to studies of interaction. It tells us, for example, that an interrogative sentence is not always used to carry out the function of requesting information but can also be used to request that an action be carried out (e.g. *Can you turn off the television please?*) or to express surprise (e.g. *Can you believe that?*). Further, it tells us that we can expect other syntactic forms, such as declarative sentences, to function as requests for information in certain contexts (e.g. *I wonder when that school was built*). In fact, in looking through the speech act literature, one might get the idea that chaos reigns in language use – that each form has a multitude of possible functions and that each function has a multitude of possible forms which can fulfill it. Fortunately, this situation is to a large extent an artifact of the methodology of speech act theorists, who, according to Goffman's term (1981: 32), are guilty of the "sins of noncontextuality." Much of the ambiguity regarding the functions of utterances isolated from context is actually done away with in real-life communicative situations. According to Schegloff (1978), this process of disambiguation is so natural that most of the time interlocutors do not even realize that the context has cleared up any ambiguity of the utterance they are hearing.

Given that the interactions which serve as the data base for the present study are laden with comprehension and production problems, I have found it advantageous to begin with grammatical and sequential rather than contextual definitions of question and response pairs. This means defining as a question (1) utterances in which the finite verb is placed in front of the subject (Did *you make this bracelet?*, *I got that out*, did*n't I?*); (2) utterances in which a wh-word is in the initial position (Who *gave you those?*); and (3) utterances with rising "question" intonation whose syntactic form is either that of a statement or a sentence fragment as illustrated by examples 1 and 2. Prior to example 1 Elsie's attempts to drink water directly from a glass resulted in spilling a good deal of the water. I was, therefore, trying to get Elsie to drink the water with the help of a straw, which she apparently did not remember how to do.

Example 1

ELSIE: I don't know just exactly.
HEIDI: You don't know how to do that? Here. Let's try it without
the straw.

((13) July 12, 1985)

The declarative question (term used by Quirk, Greenbaum, Leech, and Svartvik 1972: 392), *You don't know how to do that?*, is identical in form to the statement, *You don't know how to do that*, except for its final rising question intonation. It serves simultaneously to expand Elsie's statement and to request confirmation from Elsie of my interpretation of what she has just said.

In example 2, Elsie and I are looking at a mail-order catalogue she is carrying around the health care center with her. Because of the nonspecific nature of Elsie's utterances, I am uncertain what she means by *the most*.

Example 2

ELSIE: Now this is something here. So now which is the most?
        Does that look like that is?
HEIDI: The most things to order? The most books here?

((11) March 17, 1984

My responses to her questions are in the form of sentence fragments (*The most things to order, The most books here*) which contain no finite verb, but are uttered with final rising question intonation. These fragments simultaneously offer alternative interpretations and seek confirmation of one of those interpretations from Elsie.

My decision to work with a grammatical definition of questions excludes contextually defined "questions" from my analysis. These declarative sentences (e.g. *I wonder when that school was built*) seem to be defined as "questions" only with reference to the response they receive; that is, if they receive a response that normally would be received by a question (e.g. *I think 1965*), they are identified as questions; if they do not receive such a response (e.g. *Me too*, or no response at all), they can be identified as carrying out some other act in conversation. Given this situation where a response determines the function of the utterance which elicits it, how would I be able to assess the appropriateness of response? For example, if Elsie did not respond to a declarative sentence, such as *I wonder where that book went*, that sentence would not be defined as a question but as a statement used to convey information about the speaker; if she did respond, however, with information about the location of the book, the sentence would be defined as a question. Since initial observations of the data indicate that Elsie often does not respond to interrogative sentences requesting information or action, it does not seem sensible to have her potentially inappropriate behavior driving the identification of a given utterance as a question or not. Considering the degree of comprehension and production problems in the conversations under study, it seems to be more straightforward to work with grammatically defined questions (which may fulfill a variety of functions) and sequentially defined responses than to attempt to determine what may or may not function as a question or a response in a given situation.

Analyses

The analyses of questions and responses in this study were carried out on the conversations which took place between Elsie and me on March 5, 1982, September 5, 1982, March 17, 1984, July 12, 1985, and March 18,

1986. These five conversations selected from among the fourteen conversations in the corpus are lengthy conversations which represent different phases of Alzheimer's disease. In the course of the five conversations, 598 questions are asked – 217 by Elsie and 381 by me. The fact that these five conversations comprise 60.2% of the total speaking time (2 hours and 39 minutes of a total 4 hours and 24 minutes) and contain 59.7% of the total questions asked (598 of 1002) indicates that the distribution of questions in these conversations is representative of the entire corpus.

In preparation for the analysis of the appropriateness of responses to these questions, it was found that some of the 598 questions had to be discarded. Since, as we will see in the next chapter, one of the ways in which a question can be responded to inappropriately is not to be responded to at all, I had to be as certain as I could be that the reason for any non-response was not difficulty in hearing the question. A question was, therefore, discarded from further analysis if, because of simultaneous talk on the part of both participants, the question was apparently not heard and therefore not responded to. This situation is illustrated in example 3, in which I respond to Elsie's first question with "Mhm," but continue to talk ("Oh this is interesting") throughout her second question ("Isn't that good?").

> *Example 3*
>
> ELSIE: You've seen (the ones and) the other places,
>   too, ⌜ haven't you? ⌜ Isn't that good?
> HEIDI: └ Mhm.   └ Mhm. Oh this is interesting.
> ELSIE: Sure. Yeah.
>
> ((6) March 5, 1982)

Further, I had to be as certain as I could be that the reason for any non-response was not due to the fact that the speaker gave the conversational partner no time to respond, but instead followed immediately with a reformulation of the question or even an answer to her own question. Example 4 illustrates this situation, in which I am thwarted in my efforts to respond to Elsie's series of questions because she continues to talk herself.

> *Example 4*
>
> ELSIE: Where do you think we want to go? Go
>   outdoors? ⌜ And do a little work? I don't know.
> HEIDI: └ I don't
> ELSIE: It may be pretty cold.
>
> ((6) March 5, 1982)

Additionally, because the analyses regarding the appropriateness of responses to these questions are restricted to Elsie's and my responses to each other's questions, the few questions which were addressed by Elsie or me to a third party, such as to a health care center resident walking by, were also discarded. This situation is illustrated in example 5.

Example 5

RESIDENT: (She was dusting the room)
ELSIE: What?
HEIDI: She what?
RESIDENT: She's dusting the room (after) I go to bed.

((11) March 17, 1984)

Finally, if a response to a given question was not acoustically or articulatorily discernible to the degree necessary to carry out the appropriateness evaluation as described in the next chapter, it was discarded. In example 6, I am unable to hear Elsie's response to my request for clarification (*You do what?*) despite repeated listening to the tape, although my utterance following hers (*Yeah*) indicates that I could hear it at the time.

Example 6

HEIDI: Hi, Elsie. Hi there. ⌐ Hi [kisses Elsie].
ELSIE: ⌐ [chuckles]   [chuckles]
HEIDI: Good to see you.
ELSIE: [chuckles] I do ( )
HEIDI: You do what?
ELSIE: ( )
HEIDI: Yeah.

((13) July 12, 1985)

In what follows, I present findings of analyses in the following areas: (1) relative percentages of the total number of questions asked over time; (2) relative percentages of (grammatical) question types asked over time; (3) differential use of various wh-questions; (4) temporal and spatial reference in questions; and (5) functions of questions. In these analyses, I examine not only Elsie's use of questions, but mine as well. This comparison allows us to identify some interesting similarities and differences in our communicative behaviors. More compelling, however, than the specific findings, which could be expected to vary according to a variety of contextual factors, are the interactional trends discovered upon close examination of these findings. These interactional trends are discussed with reference to

Table 1. *Relative percentages of questions asked by Elsie and Heidi in five selected conversations*

(no. = 518; actual number of questions in parentheses)

	Heidi	Elsie	Totals
March 1982	43% (44)	57% (59)	103
September 1982	43% (49)	57% (66)	115
March 1984	63% (66)	37% (39)	105
July 1985	93% (110)	7% (8)	118
March 1986	96% (74)	4% (3)	77
Average	66% (343)	34% (175)	518

the framework of division of labor in discourse outlined above. Within that framework, adjustments in my questioning behavior are seen as "before-the-fact" measures to compensate for Elsie's behavior (or what I perceive this to be) on the levels of proportion of questions asked; (grammatical) types of questions asked; temporal and spatial reference; and question function.

Proportion of total number of questions

An examination of the 518 questions across the five conversations, as seen in table 1, reveals that Elsie's part in asking questions becomes smaller and smaller over time, beginning with 57% of the questions asked in March 1982 and ending with 4% four years later in March of 1986, the largest single drop-off in percentage occurring between the March 1984 conversation and the conversation in July 1985 (37% to 7%).

Accordingly, as Elsie's proportion of questions becomes increasingly smaller, my proportion becomes increasingly greater, beginning with 43% of the questions asked in March of 1982 and ending with 96% in March of 1986. This information suggests that as Elsie becomes increasingly unable or unwilling over time to use questions to initiate new topics and to follow up on current ones, I take over a greater share of discourse work by producing an increasing proportion of the total number of questions in our interactions. From an interactional perspective, however, in which *both* conversational partners are responsible for the configuration of the conversations, it is important to keep in mind throughout this discussion the possibility that I am (for some reason) becoming an increasingly assertive interlocutor who is, in a sense, edging Elsie out of the conversations.

It is interesting to compare this indication of Elsie's and my relative

Table 2. *Number of words produced by both
conversational partners*

(percentages of total number of words given in parentheses)

	Heidi	Elsie
March 1982 (41 mins.)	1,733 (27%)	4,639 (73%)
Sept. 1982 (31 mins.)	1,605 (31%)	3,625 (69%)
March 1984 (38 mins.)	1,077 (20%)	4,336 (80%)
July 1985 (26 mins.)	1,224 (72%)	467 (28%)
March 1986 (23 mins.)	683 (88%)	91 (12%)

involvement in these conversations in terms of questioning activity with
our overall participation in each conversation as represented by a simple
count of words uttered, as seen in table 2.

Combining the information on Elsie's relative degree of participation in
these five conversations as gleaned from tables 1 and 2, we can provide the
following preliminary characterizations of three different stages in the
patient's discourse production, at least as it plays out in these interactions.
We shall return to these characterizations in the next two chapters, where
additional relevant findings will be incorporated to provide a more
elaborated picture of the stages.

The first two conversations are characterized by a high level of patient
participation in terms both of percentage of total number of words
produced and percentage of total number of questions asked. The third
conversation is characterized by a continued high level of patient participation in conversation in terms of percentage of total number of words
produced but a somewhat lower patient participation in conversation in
terms of percentage of total number of questions asked when compared
with the first two conversations. The final two conversations are characterized by a substantially reduced level of patient participation in conversation, both in terms of percentage of total number of words produced
and in terms of percentage of total number of questions asked when
compared with the first three conversations. This characterization of Elsie
in the final two conversations as having a substantially reduced level of
participation is corroborated by a study of ten late-stage Alzheimer's
patients by Causino, Obler, Knoefel, and Albert (forthcoming) in which
they observe the "nondemented conversational partner bearing most of
the weight of the conversation," as they put it. Their subjects seldom
initiated or did anything to prolong the conversations.

At first blush, it is tempting to interpret Elsie's decreasing production of
questions over time as evidence of decreasing communicative initiative on

her part – that she is becoming more withdrawn and less willing and able to engage in the kind of intersubjectivity which question-asking necessarily entails. The situation, however, is not that simple. We must take into account the *functions* which the questions are being used to fulfill. For example, the use of a question to request information or to request action arguably shows more initiative on the speaker's part than the use of a question to check one's understanding of what the other person just said, although each of these functions intrinsically indicates an interest to move the interaction along. As we shall see later in the discussion of question functions, Elsie did continue to ask more questions to request information than to do anything else in conversation up until our conversation in March 1986.

Percentage of question types

Each of the 518 questions was examined to determine the question type it represents. In addition to the yes–no questions, wh-questions, and alternative questions discussed above, question types in this study include *okay?* which serves to check the conversational partner's agreement or comprehension, as well as signals of an acoustic problem (*huh?, hmm?*). The final two question types, in contrast to the first three, work to ensure that what Goffman (1981: 12) calls the "very fundamental requirements of talk as a communication system" are fulfilled. *Okay?* helps a speaker to find out whether his or her message has been received; a signal of an acoustic problem such as *hmm?* helps a listener to show that he or she has not received the message. Example 7 illustrates a yes–no question I ask Elsie.

Example 7

HEIDI: Is that when you quit working?
ELSIE: Uh::. I don't remember.

((8) May 20, 1982)

Example 8 illustrates a wh-question Elsie asks me.

Example 8

ELSIE: Where are we going?
HEIDI: We're going to exercise class.

((2) November 20, 1981)

Table 3. *Relative percentages of types of questions asked by Elsie and Heidi in five selected conversations*

(real numbers in parentheses)

		Wh-questions	Yes–No questions	huh?/hmm?	Okay?	alternative	Totals
3/82	Heidi	14% (6)	82% (36)	0%	0%	4% (2)	44
	Elsie	22% (13)	69% (41)	7% (4)	0%	2% (1)	59
9/82	Heidi	31% (13)	62% (32)	0%	8% (4)	0%	49
	Elsie	24% (16)	74% (49)	2% (1)	0%	0%	66
3/84	Heidi	39% (26)	52% (34)	5% (3)	5% (3)	0%	66
	Elsie	13% (5)	74% (29)	13% (5)	0%	0%	39
7/85	Heidi	8% (9)	69% (76)	9% (10)	14% (15)	0%	110
	Elsie	63% (5)	37% (3)	0%	0%	0%	8
3/86	Heidi	8% (6)	78% (58)	8% (6)	5% (4)	0%	74
	Elsie	0%	0%	100% (3)	0%	0%	3
AVG:	Heidi	17% (60)	69% (236)	6% (19)	8% (26)	1% (2)	343
	Elsie	22% (39)	70% (122)	7% (13)	0%	1% (1)	175

Example 9 illustrates an alternative question I ask Elsie.

> *Example 9*
>
> HEIDI: <u>Do you want me to help you move</u>
> <u>over there or do you want to sit</u>
> <u>by the window?</u>⌐
> ELSIE: ⌐ No. I guess. Oh.
> How did you do that? You mean slow this one?
>
>   ((6) March 5, 1982)

Only three alternative questions were asked during the five selected conversations – one by Elsie and two by me.

Example 10 illustrates my use of *okay?* to check Elsie's agreement/comprehension.

> *Example 10*
>
> HEIDI: I'll come back to see you next week.
> <u>Okay?</u> You said you wanted me to,
> so I'll do it.⌐
> ELSIE: ⌐ Mhm.
>
>   ((13) July 12, 1985)

Example 11 shows Elsie signaling an acoustic problem through the use of *huh?*

Example 11

HEIDI: That's an order blank.
ELSIE: Huh?
HEIDI: That's an order blank. ⌜ If you want to
ELSIE: ⌞ Oh I see.
HEIDI: buy some of these things then you write them down and send this in.
ELSIE: Oh yes. I see.

((11) March 17, 1984)

Regarding Elsie's and my average use of the various question types over the five conversations, we note in table 3 that of the 518 questions asked, yes–no questions are more frequent than wh-questions for both Elsie and me.

Differential use of various wh-questions

Because of the relatively small number of wh-questions (39 by Elsie; 60 by me) among the 518 questions from five selected conversations, I examined the wh-questions in all fourteen conversations. Because it has been discussed in the literature that Alzheimer's patients are context-bound (Obler 1981; Appell, Kertesz, and Fisman 1982) and use a great deal of automatic speech (Bayles and Kaszniak 1987), I wanted to examine in greater detail the *what* questions and the *how* questions. One hypothesis was that Elsie, if she were truly context-bound, would produce more *what*-questions which refer to concrete objects in the "here and now" than those which refer to objects not in the physical environment or to actions. Further, because of the documented use of automatic language by Alzheimer's patients, I hypothesized that a greater percentage of Elsie's *how*-questions would be *How are you?* than all other nonformulaic uses involving *how*.

Example 12 illustrates the use of a *what*-question to refer to a concrete object in the "here and how," i.e. something in Elsie's bag.

Example 12

HEIDI: What do you have in here?
ELSIE: I'm gonna try to get another in it. Oh no. It's a lotta ( ) (stamps).

((8) May 20, 1982)

Table 4. *Hierarchy of wh-question words used by*
Heidi and Elsie in all conversations

(number of occurrences in parentheses)

Heidi	no. = 119	Elsie	no. = 112
what-concrete	34% (40)	where	38% (43)
what-other	32% (38)	what-other	22% (25)
how-formula	13% (15)	which	10% (11)
where	8% (10)	how-other	9% (10)
who	6% (7)	what-concrete	7% (8)
which	5% (6)	how-formula	5% (6)
how-other	2% (2)	when	4% (5)
why	1% (1)	why	3% (3)
when	0% (0)	who	1% (1)

Example 13 illustrates the other group of *what*-questions which refers to objects not in the physical environment.

Example 13

ELSIE: What street?
HEIDI: I live on Walter Road.

((10) October 2, 1982)

Example 14 illustrates a *what*-question which refers to an action rather than to a concrete object.

Example 14

HEIDI: What're you doing?
ELSIE: Oh, I'm getting things .. gettin some things (cleanin up).

((8) May 20, 1982)

As noted above, *how*-questions were also separated into two groups. One group refers to a formulaic question involving the wh-word *how*, as illustrated by example 15.

Example 15

ELSIE: How are you?
HEIDI: I'm fine.

((8) May 20, 1982)

The other group of *how*-questions refers to all other nonformulaic uses involving *how*, one of which is illustrated by example 16.

Example 16

ELSIE: How'd we get here all of a sudden?
HEIDI: I don't know.

((7) May 18, 1982)

The results of this analysis are presented in table 4.

According to the findings in table 4, not only are both hypotheses incorrect for Elsie's question production, they fit *my own* question production. Whereas only 7% of Elsie's wh-questions were about concrete objects, 34% of mine fit this category. More of Elsie's *what*-questions refer to actions or objects not in the environment than refer to concrete objects. Additionally, the formulaic expression *how are you*? comprises only 5% of Elsie's wh-questions. She uses *how* more frequently in newly created questions than in formulaic questions. On the other hand, the formulaic expression comprises 13% of my wh-questions, whereas only 2% of my wh-questions contain *how* in a non-formulaic question.

It appears that I am designing my utterances to fit my *perceptions* of Elsie's communicative and cognitive abilities. Thinking that she is most able to talk about concrete objects, I ask her more questions about such objects in the environment. Thinking that she is most able to engage successfully in formulaic question/response pairs, I pose more such questions of her. However, Elsie's relatively less frequent use of formulaic questions and questions regarding concrete objects suggest that my perceptions of her abilities do not match reality. In their examination of accommodation and healthy elderly individuals, Coupland, Coupland, Giles, and Henwood (1988) suggest that younger speakers may regularly *overaccommodate* their speech to these elderly individuals. This over-accommodation occurs, they suggest, because the younger speakers "are accommodating *not* to individuals' communicative characteristics *per se*, but rather, to those they stereotype the elderly as possessing" (1988: 9). In a later study, Coupland, Coupland, and Grainger (1991: 192) found that linguistic choices made by younger conversational partners in intergenerational conversations actually help to construct "elderly" identities for the older interlocutors. The mismatches observed above turn my attempts at accommodation into overaccommodation. This greater amount of talk about the concrete environment and involving formulaic exchanges than would have been necessary may serve to co-construct a "patient" identity for Elsie.

Spatial and temporal reference in questions

Elsie's and my yes–no questions, wh-questions, and alternative questions were also examined to determine spatial and temporal reference. Tokens of *okay?* and *hmm?* were disregarded in this analysis because they do not refer to an event, object, or person in time and space, but fulfill a more mechanical function in conversation.

Spatial reference: First, I determined the spatial reference of each of the yes–no questions, wh-questions, and alternative questions. In this study, if the question refers to events, objects, or persons within sight, its spatial reference is proximal. If the question refers to events, objects, or persons outside the range of sight, its spatial reference is distal. Example 17 illustrates a question with proximal reference. At this point in the interaction, Elsie and I are talking immediately following the exercise class about how much we enjoy it.

Example 17

ELSIE: We have a good time, don't we?
HEIDI: Yes we do. We sure do.

((4) November 25, 1981)

In this example, Elsie is referring to events and/or a state of mind which are anchored to the current location.

Example 18 illustrates a question with distal reference.

Example 18

HEIDI: Is that when you quit working?
ELSIE: Uh::. I don't remember.

((8) May 20, 1982)

In this question, I am referring not only to a distant time but also to a distant place in Elsie's life.

When we look at the individual conversations as represented in table 5, we see that from March 1984 onward, Elsie uses proximal reference *exclusively*. (In March 1986, Elsie only produces three tokens of *hmm?*.) An examination of my use of spatial reference shows a continual increase over time in proximal reference, beginning with 64% (28 of 44) proximal reference in March 1982 and ending with 98% (63 of 64) proximal reference four years later. Against the backdrop of division of labor in discourse, then, it is likely that my continuing increase of proximal reference over the five conversations is in response to what I perceive to be Elsie's difficulty in making reference to distant persons, objects, and events. In noting a deficiency in the type of discourse work which Elsie can carry out, I respond accordingly.

Temporal reference: Next I examined each question to determine whether its temporal referent is located in the remote past, recent past, present, near future, or distant future. In this study, recent past refers to times earlier in the same day; remote past refers to the previous day and farther back in time. The near future refers to times later in the same day; distant future refers to the next day and beyond.

Example 19 illustrates reference to the remote past. In this interaction, Elsie and I are looking at some of her belongings in her room. I see an original oil painting on the wall and ask Elsie the following question.

Example 19

HEIDI: Did you do that?
ELSIE: I don't .. I didn't but my brother I think did.

((9) September 5, 1982)

Since it is quite obvious that the picture was not painted earlier that day, my question refers to the remote past in its attempt to find out if Elsie is the artist.

Example 20 illustrates reference to the recent past.

Example 20

HEIDI: Did you have your lunch yet?
ELSIE: mhm

((13) July 12, 1985)

Example 21 illustrates reference to the present time. In this interaction, Elsie is sitting in the lounge next to some large picture windows on a cool March day.

Example 21

ELSIE: My, it's quite cool, ⌐isn't it?
HEIDI: └Yes it is. I think it's probably cool because you're right next to the window there.

((6) March 5, 1982)

Example 22 illustrates reference to the near future. Just prior to this segment, I told Elsie that we are going to have an ice cream party in the afternoon.

Table 5. *Spatial reference used by Elsie and Heidi in five selected conversations*

(no. = 460)

	Elsie's questions (no. = 162)			Heidi's questions (no. = 298)		
	Proximal	Distal	Totals	Proximal	Distal	Totals
3/82	84% (46)	16% (9)	55	64% (28)	36% (16)	44
9/82	72% (47)	28% (18)	65	78% (35)	22% (10)	45
3/84	100% (34)	0%	34	88% (53)	12% (7)	60
7/85	100% (8)	0%	8	94% (80)	6% (5)	85
3/86	0%	0%	0	98% (63)	2% (1)	64
AVG:	83% (135)	17% (27)	162	87% (259)	13% (39)	298

Example 22

ELSIE: Oh, we'll stay right ⌐here then,
HEIDI: ⌐Yeah.
ELSIE: won't we?
HEIDI: Uhhuh. Yeah.

((3) November 20, 1981)

Here Elsie is checking her understanding of what she should do in the afternoon, i.e. stay right in the lounge on her floor and wait to be picked up and taken to the party.

Example 23 illustrates reference to the distant future. In this segment, I am preparing to leave Elsie for the day.

Example 23

HEIDI: Would you like me to come next week to see you?
ELSIE: Sure. Sure.

((13) July 12, 1985)

This is the only instance of reference to the future beyond the present day in all five conversations. And, even here, one could make the argument that this example does not really refer to some future action but to Elsie's current wishes.

Tables 6 and 7 indicate the temporal reference of Elsie's and my questions during the five selected conversations. Since, during these five conversations, Elsie never makes reference to the distant future, and I

Table 6. *Temporal reference used by Elsie in five selected conversations*

(no. = 162)

	Remote past	Recent past	Present	Near future	Totals
3/82	11% (6)	22% (12)	62% (34)	5% (3)	55
9/82	8% (5)	26% (17)	57% (37)	9% (6)	65
3/84	0%	9% (3)	76% (26)	15% (5)	34
7/85	0%	12% (1)	88% (7)	0%	8
3/86	0%	0%	0%	0%	0
AVG:	7% (11)	20% (33)	64% (104)	9% (14)	162

Table 7. *Temporal reference used by Heidi in five selected conversations*

(no. = 297/ one instance of reference to remote future in 7/85 not represented in table)

	Remote past	Recent past	Present	Near future	Totals
3/82	27% (12)	14% (6)	50% (22)	9% (4)	44
9/82	27% (12)	0%	69% (31)	4% (2)	45
3/84	13% (8)	3% (2)	82% (49)	2% (1)	60
7/85	5% (4)	5% (4)	88% (75)	1% (1)	84
3/86	6% (4)	3% (2)	91% (58)	0%	64
AVG:	13% (40)	5% (14)	79% (235)	3% (8)	297

make reference to it only once, this temporal category does not appear in these tables.

As we see in tables 6 and 7, over the five conversations Elsie actually refers *less* on average to the present time questions than I do (64% (104 of 162) vs. 79% (235 of 298) (p < 0.01). Only in our conversation of March 1982 does Elsie refer more to the present time than I do. The percentage of my questions which refers to the present time steadily increases from 50% in March 1982 up to 91% in March 1986. With the exception of our conversation in September 1982, Elsie also tends to refer increasingly to the present time.

Of the greater proportion of Elsie's questions which refer to the past and the future, 9% (14 of 162) of Elsie's questions refer to the (near) future, as compared with only 3% (8 of 298) of mine. Twenty-seven percent (44 of 162) of Elsie's questions refer to the past as compared with only 18% (54 of 298) of mine. When we look more closely at Elsie's and my reference to the past, however, we note that I refer more often to the remote past, whereas Elsie refers more often to the recent past.

Just as we observed earlier in our discussion of the production of wh-questions what may be interpreted as overaccommodation on my part to Elsie's abilities, here again it appears that I am designing my utterances to fit my *perception* of Elsie's communicative and cognitive abilities. Thinking that she is more capable of talking about the present time, I talk more about the present time. Thinking that she is incapable of projecting into the future, or incapable of remembering the past, I do not often question what will happen in the future or what has happened in the past. However, Elsie's relatively greater reference to the future and the past suggest that my perceptions of her abilities do not match reality and that, as the healthy interlocutor, I influence the greater amount of talk about the present time than would have been necessary.

Functions of questions

Finally, each question (including the instances of *okay?* and *hmm?* which were excluded in the reference analyses) was examined to determine its primary function in the discourse. The questions were found to fulfill the following functions: requesting information, requesting action, checking one's own understanding (or indicating one's own problems in understanding), exclaiming, checking the other's understanding/agreement, and testing/tutoring.

Example 24 illustrates a question which functions as a request for information. Prior to this segment I have just given Elsie another drink of water and am preparing to leave for the day.

Example 24

ELSIE: What is this day?
HEIDI: What is today? It's Friday. It's Friday today. Friday, July 12, 1985.

((13) July 12, 1985)

In this example, I understand Elsie's question (*What is this day?*) to be requesting information either about the day of the week or the calendar date. In my response I give her both pieces of information.

Example 25 illustrates a question which functions as a request for action. Elsie is lying in bed and I bring a copy of the *National Geographic* magazine to her and ask the following question.

Example 25

HEIDI: Want to open it up and look at it a little bit? Let's see what's in here.

((14) March 18, 1986)

In this example, my question serves as a request for Elsie to open up the magazine.

Example 26 illustrates a question which functions to check the speaker's understanding of the previous utterance. In this segment, Elsie and I are walking from the elevators to the lounge on the second floor. We have just passed the nurses' station which was decorated with turkeys for the Thanksgiving holiday.

Example 26

HEIDI: Did you see the turkeys?
ELSIE: <u>Oh here you mean?</u> ┌<u>Right there?</u>
HEIDI: └Yeah. Yeah.

((4) November 25, 1981)

Elsie uses her questions (*Oh here you mean?* and *Right there?*) to check that she has understood my question as I had intended it to be understood.

Example 27 illustrates a question which functions as an exclamation. In this segment, Elsie and I are standing at the window in her room looking outside. Elsie sees the colorful flag blowing in the wind.

Example 27

ELSIE: Look at all the colors. ┌<u>Aren't they</u>
HEIDI: └Mhm.
ELSIE: <u>pretty?</u> ┐
HEIDI: └ Yeah.
ELSIE: I should say so.

((6) March 5, 1982)

In this example, Elsie uses a question to exclaim about the beauty of the colors she sees.

Example 28 illustrates a question which functions to test or tutor the conversational partner. The defining characteristic of such questions is that, although they look like requests for information, the speaker already knows the answer. In this segment, Elsie and I are talking about our previous residence in the Midwestern United States.

Table 8. *Functions fulfilled by Elsie's questions in five selected conversations*
(no. = 175)

	request information	check own under- standing	request action	exclaim	tutorial	check other's under- standing	totals
3/82	47% (28)	34% (20)	2% (1)	17% (10)	0%	0%	59
9/82	62% (41)	23% (15)	6% (4)	9% (6)	0%	0%	66
3/84	74% (29)	18% (7)	5% (2)	3% (1)	0%	0%	39
7/85	63% (5)	37% (3)	0	0%	0%	0%	8
3/86	0%	100% (3)	0	0%	0%	0%	3
AVG:	59% (103)	27% (48)	4% (7)	10% (17)	0%	0%	175

Example 28

HEIDI: And I lived for the last two years in
 Minnesota, ┌ so I w
ELSIE: └ Yeah so do I.
HEIDI: Uhhuh.
ELSIE: That's ┌ where I was born, ┌ too.
HEIDI: └ uhhuh uhhuh   └ uhhuh. You
were down in Mankato? ┐
ELSIE: └ Yes. Mhm.

((6) March 5, 1982)

In this example, I use the question *You were down in Mankato?* to help
provide Elsie with information to continue our conversation. Because I
know the answer is affirmative, I can be seen as either tutoring or testing
her.

Example 29 illustrates *okay?* functioning to check the conversational
partner's understanding of or agreement with what was just said. Just
prior to this segment, I have gone to the nurses' station to get a straw
which I think will help Elsie drink some water from a glass. Upon my
return I say the following.

Example 29

HEIDI: Here you go. Here you go. Let's try
 to drink it this way. Okay?
ELSIE: Sure.

((13) July 12, 1985)

Table 9. *Functions fulfilled by Heidi's questions in five selected conversations*

(no. = 343)

	request information	check own under-standing	request action	exclaim	tutorial	check other's under-standing	totals
3/82	66% (29)	20% (9)	0%	7% (3)	7% (3)	0%	44
9/82	67% (33)	10% (5)	8% (4)	6% (3)	0%	8% (4)	49
3/84	35% (23)	53% (35)	1% (1)	1% (1)	5% (3)	5% (3)	66
7/85	42% (46)	25% (28)	15% (16)	3% (3)	2% (2)	14% (15)	110
3/86	49% (36)	14% (10)	15% (11)	8% (6)	9% (7)	5% (4)	74
AVG:	49% (167)	25% (87)	9% (32)	5% (16)	4% (15)	8% (26)	343

In this example, I am using *okay?* to elicit Elsie's agreement for what I suggested in my previous utterance, i.e. that she should try to drink the water through a straw.

Tables 8 and 9 show us that, on average, both Elsie and I ask proportionately more questions to request information than to fulfill any other function. Fifty-nine percent (103 of 175) of Elsie's questions are requests for information; 49% (167 of 343) of my questions fulfill that function. Elsie continues to ask proportionately more questions to request information than to check her own understanding up until the very last conversation in our sample in March 1986. Even in July 1985, when she asks only 7% of total questions in the conversation, she still asks more questions to request information (63%: 5 of 8) than to check her understanding (37%: 3 of 8). The second most frequent function our questions serve to fulfill is to check our own understanding of what the other person has just said. On average, 27% (48 of 175) of Elsie's questions are of this type; 25% (87 of 343) of mine fulfill this function. As noted in the discussion of other-initiated repairs in chapter 2, however, Elsie uses only nonspecific requests for repetition (e.g. *huh?*) in our conversations in 1985 and 1986.

In March 1984, in contrast to the other four conversations, a greater proportion of my questions are used to check my own understanding than to request information from Elsie (53% vs. 35%). This situation makes sense when we consider that in March 1984 Elsie still is producing a great deal of language (unlike the following two conversations, see table 2) but this language is increasingly incoherent, causing me to respond frequently with follow-up questions in an attempt to ensure that I am understanding what Elsie is saying.

In the final two conversations we note a substantial increase in the percentage of the questions I use to request an action from Elsie (*Can you sit up a little more?, Can you drink some?,* and *Can you suck on the straw?*). In July 1985 as well as in March 1986, 15% (16 of 110 and 11 of 74, respectively) of my questions fulfill this function. This stands in contrast to no occurrences in March 1982, 8% (4 of 49) in September 1982, and 1% (1 of 66) in March 1984. It appears that my questions were being used increasingly less in *verbal* interchanges (such as would be precipitated by the use of a question to request information) and more in situations where an appropriate response to a question could be an *action* rather than a verbal response. For example, when I ask Elsie, *Can you suck on the straw?* an appropriate response would not need to include the verbal response *yes* or *no*, but could be an attempt to put her lips to the straw or a deliberate pushing away of the straw. My use of a greater percentage of such questions at a time when Elsie's overall linguistic production is diminished serves as a successful means of carrying on a "dialogue" – albeit a dialogue comprised of verbal questions and nonverbal (action) responses. On the other hand, during these same two conversations, Elsie uses no questions to request an action on my part. This contrasts with the small but consistent proportion of her questions (2%, 6%, and 5%) used to fulfill this function during the first three conversations.

During the final two conversations, Elsie produces not one question with an exclamatory function (e.g. *Isn't that pretty?*). An examination of the first three conversations shows a decreasing trend in Elsie's use of this type of question, from 17% (10 of 59) of her total questions in March 1982 to 9% (6 of 66) in September 1982 to only 3% (1 of 39) in March 1984. This evidence may support the presentation of Elsie as an increasingly less active verbal communicator. The exclamatory function arguably contributes less to the overall conversation than functions which ensure that the conversation continues to be fueled with new ideas and actions, and that the mechanical requirements of the conversation are met. We can speculate that this exclamatory function is the first to go as more effort is needed to communicate, allowing Elsie to expend her limited conversational energy on idea-producing functions or ultimately on mechanically important functions which indicate that the other's utterance was not heard well enough to answer.

Summary and implications

This chapter provided information on Elsie's use of questions in five selected conversations between March 1982 and March 1986 as compared with mine. Here we observed that (1) Elsie produced an increasingly smaller proportion of the total number of questions in our conversations over time, ranging from 57% in March 1982 to only 4% four years later; (2) Elsie used a greater number of yes–no questions (70%) than wh-questions (22%) on average across the five conversations; (3) Elsie used "where" and "what" most frequently of all wh-question words (they comprised a total of 67% of Elsie's wh-questions); (4) Elsie used a greater percentage of proximal spatial reference (83% proximal; 17% distal), and from March 1984 onward made exclusive use of proximal reference; (5) Elsie referred more frequently to the present time (64%) than to the past (27%) or the future (9%); and (5) Elsie used questions most frequently to serve as requests for information (59%), followed by checks of her own understanding (27%).

My own question production was then explained within the framework of division of labor in discourse where we saw a variety of instances of what appears to be compensation (or overcompensation) to what I perceived to be Elsie's difficulties in discourse. For example, as Elsie produced fewer questions, I produced more over time. As she referred more (and later exclusively) to our present location, I increasingly did so, too (from 64% in March 1982 to 98% four years later). As she became less able to respond verbally to my questions, I produced more questions which could have nonverbal action as an appropriate response. On several occasions, it appeared that my preconceptions of Elsie's abilities did not match her actual production, possibly influencing me to refer more to the present time (79% vs. 64%) as well as to concrete objects (34% vs. 7%) than Elsie did.

As a result of these analyses, I believe there are two important warnings regarding research into communication between "normal" and "communicatively disabled" conversationalists. First, the cases we examined above provide evidence that I, as the "normal" partner, am accommodating to what I *perceive* to be Elsie's communicative and cognitive capabilities but which appear not to match Elsie's actual abilities. This situation urges us strongly to analyze not only the communicative behavior of the disabled participant, but of *all* participants, in an interaction. As we have seen, it could very well be the preconceptions of the "normal" partner (e.g. therapist, health-care provider, or family member) which are influencing the topics talked about by the patient and even the grammatical categories used by the patient to talk about them. If the influence of the healthy conversational partner is not recognized, the danger exists that various labels can be forced onto the patient's communicative abilities which are not suitable in and of themselves, or at least not to the extent imagined. Coupland, Coupland, and Grainger (1991: 207) point out that interactional factors such as these must be seen as contributing to the social construction of the individuals' identities within the discourse itself. Although they are talking about healthy aging, their points are valid for the construction of the patient's identities as well. "A shift of attention from a demographic category treated as an isolated sociolingusitic variable to talk as a mode of action between humans of varying situational identities, allows us to develop a much richer understanding of how discourse helps us to construct the fabric of social life in ageing." In short, it is necessary to take into account any other persons involved in an interaction with a "communicatively disabled" person, so as to attain the most precise information possible regarding the disabled individual's communicative abilities and disabilities.

Second, we must be careful to provide justification for any different interpretation we give a phenomenon used by a disabled individual as opposed to that we give a phenomenon used by a "normal" individual. It is all too easy to say that, if a given phenomenon is used by a patient, it reflects the pathology, whereas if it is used by the "normal" person, it is "accommodation" to the patient or part of an attempt to save face. For example, in examining Elsie's and my questions to find evidence for Elsie's context-boundedness, we find evidence which would suggest that *I* am the one who is context-bound, since I refer on average more than Elsie does to concrete objects, and to the present time and place. In their examinations of Alzheimer's patients in conversations with a healthy partner as compared with healthy elderly in conversations with the same healthy partner, Ripich, Vertes, Whitehouse, Fulton, and Ekelman (1991) observe that the Alzheimer's patients use assertives less than healthy elderly individuals do. They interpret this difference as suggesting "a lack of awareness or concern regarding their own [the Alzheimer's patients'] opinions. It could also be interpreted as a lack of confidence in their own thinking." But when one examines the tables accompanying the article, one finds that the healthy examiner uses even fewer assertives than the Alzheimer's patients do. If the discourse behavior of the examiner were to be interpreted in the same light as that of the research subjects, we would have to say that she has even less awareness of her own opinions or has even less confidence in her own thinking than the Alzheimer's patients. Of course, that interpretation would be absurd. My point is not that the healthy examiner's language indicates some cognitive breakdown; the point is that we cannot responsibly decide a priori that the same linguistic phenomenon can be interpreted two different ways for two different populations without looking further for some external justification of these differential interpretations. It is likely, for example, that the examiner's behavior could be accounted for by her social role as interviewer (despite the fact that she was instructed by the researchers to talk to the subjects as peers in a conversation).

In this spirit, Campbell-Taylor (1984) seeks an explanation for the fact that account-giving (as discussed earlier in chapter 2) by Alzheimer's patients is viewed by clinicians as a marker of that disease and by laymen as "unusual behavior," when account-giving is actually a behavior used by healthy individuals. Campbell-Taylor (1984: 91) points out that this alternative interpretation of a normal behavior is probably due to the frequency with which the accounts are employed or because they were perceived as being neither effective nor sufficient.

Along this line, Tannen (1981) criticizes Labov and Fanshel (1977) for allowing knowledge of patient and therapist roles to color their interpretations of phenomena used by both participants in therapeutic interviews, resulting in the description of the therapist's talk as intentional and the patient's talk as involuntarily revealing emotions. Whereas the patient is shown to "hesitate," to "interrupt herself" and to use a "falsetto squeal," the therapist using the same linguistic devices is described as pausing, changing his approach, and using a mitigating device, respectively.

Since it seems unlikely that the "normal" conversationalist is suffering from the same cognitive and communicative breakdowns as the patient in the cases discussed above, when we encounter the same linguistic phenomena being used by both normal interlocutors and patients, we need, first, to search for quantitative and/or qualitative differences in the use of this behavior which would justify differential interpretations of it, and, barring those differences, take into account the possibility that the patient could be operating with the same motivations, such as face concerns and accommodation, as the "normal" interlocutor. Following an examination of the appropriateness of Elsie's responses to my questions over time, chapter 4 discusses one solution to this problem within the examination of response as a discourse strategy.

4 Responses

Just as every question anticipates a response, a discussion of questions without an examination of the responses to those questions would seem to dangle in midair. This examination of responses is divided into two major sections: the first on the appropriateness of Elsie's responses and the second on response as a discourse strategy.

Following a discussion of the criteria I developed to determine the appropriateness of a response in conversation, I present the results of the analysis of Elsie's responses to my questions in five selected conversations. Based on these results, I trace the qualitative changes which characterize Elsie's responses over time. In the first two conversations Elsie's inappropriateness consists primarily of vague and grammatically mismatched responses. In the third conversation, however, question type mismatches (such as *yes* responses to wh-questions) and "no responses" join the first two types of inappropriate responses in almost equal representation. In the final two conversations, Elsie's inappropriateness consists overwhelmingly in not responding to the question.

A longitudinal examination of Elsie's proportion of appropriate responses indicates no clear downward trend to accompany the progression of Alzheimer's disease. The proportion of her appropriate responses in the fourth and fifth conversations is actually higher than in the first and third conversations. The explanation of this unexpected result seems to lie in my own linguistic behavior. Analyses point to the fact that I am (unintentionally) accommodating to Elsie's changing ability to respond to various types of questions, thus enabling Elsie to continue to be a successful partner despite increasing difficulties.

The second major section of this chapter, which discusses response as a discourse strategy, begins with the findings of an analysis of my responses to Elsie's questions according to the criteria developed to analyze the appropriateness of Elsie's responses to my questions. There we are confronted with a small percentage of my responses which according to the criteria would have to be judged to be inappropriate. Further analysis of these "inappropriate" responses suggests that their design is motivated

108

by the interactional goals of coherence, positive face-maintenance, and negative face-maintenance. A model is introduced whose tridimensional space is defined by axes representing these three interactional goals and within whose space individual responses can be placed according to relative amount of focus on each goal.

Given that my "inappropriate" responses were determined to be motivated by face concerns, I then reexamine Elsie's responses which were judged to be inappropriate in the first half of the chapter in order to determine if they, too, could be understood as being "face-motivated." Subsequent analyses suggest, however, that lack of possible motivation for face concerns (as I perceived the situation at least) justify their initial determination as inappropriate responses.

Tracking the appropriateness of Elsie's responses over time

Looking towards the goal of tracking Elsie's continuing breakdown in comprehension over time, the following criteria were devised for determining the appropriateness of a response to a question. These criteria were not simply adopted from another study of responses or devised prior to or in isolation from analyses of the data under examination, but were devised based on close observation of features contained in Elsie's responses. Because these criteria *came out of* the data themselves and incorporated observations made earlier regarding Elsie's language use (e.g. structure/content dichotomy), they allow the optimal amount of *relevant* differentiation to be made among inappropriate responses. This would not have been the case, for instance, if a similar rating system from studies of first language acquisition or aphasia had been used. To illustrate this problem briefly, I have selected one study of each type.

In their study of children's comprehension of questions, Tyack and Ingram (1977) score all responses as either correct or incorrect according to standards such as the mention of an animate noun in response to a *who*-question or the mention of an inanimate noun in response to a *what*-question. This dichotomy would not have allowed me to differentiate among the types of "incorrect" responses (such as no response, change in topic, *yes* response to a wh-question, grammatical mismatch, and vague response) which I have identified in my data. In their study of comprehension in aphasics (due to left-hemisphere lesions), Boller, Cole, Vrtunski, Patterson, and Kim (1979) also score responses as correct or not, but then go on to examine if the "incorrect" responses are "appropriate" or not. By "appropriate" they mean, for example, whether the patient responded with an action of any kind to a question which requested action or with any kind of verbal response other than *yes* or *no* to a wh-question requesting information. Although the differentiation made by Boller, *et al.* between correct and appropriate is a critical one, their differentiation among "appropriate" responses is not fine-grained enough for my data.[1]

Here it is also important to remember that such definitions of discourse phenomena based on empirical data are (at least in part) culture-specific. Although some inappropriate responses, such as those which answer a wh-question with *yes* or *no*, are linguistically defective, others, such as silence or change in topic, may be inappropriate only in some cultures. Goffman (1981: 25) cites observations made by V. Hymes (1974: 9) on the Warm Springs Indian reservation in Oregon: "Unlike our norm of interaction, that at Warm Springs does not require that a question by one person be followed immediately by an answer or a promise of an answer by the addressee. It *may* be followed by an answer but *may also be followed by silence or by an utterance which bears no relationship to the question.* Then the answer to the question may follow as long as five or ten minutes later" (emphasis mine).

Before proceeding on to a discussion of my criteria for determining appropriateness of response, I would like to recognize that, by necessity, a discrete evaluation system simplifies the richness of the data judged by its criteria. It is my belief, however, that the use of this system *as a tool* (and not as an end in itself) is justified by the trends which are uncovered in Elsie's use of language, and what these trends can tell us about the effect of Alzheimer's disease on an individual's ability to communicate.

Response types

In this study, an utterance which immediately follows a question is defined as filling that question's response slot. As discussed in chapter 3, whatever follows a question is assumed by the person asking the question to be a response to the question, unless there is evidence to the contrary. Goffman (1981: 13) states: "The first pair-part [of which a question is one type] co-opts the slot that follows, indeed makes a slot out of next moments, rendering anything occurring then subject to close inspection for evidence

---

[1] Blanken, Dittmann, Haas, and Wallesch (1987) use the following response classification scheme in their examination of ten patients with moderate Alzheimer's disease as compared with Wernicke's aphasics and healthy elderly controls: (1) Fulfilling response; (2) partly-fulfilling response (fragmentary, vague, and evasive); (3) non-fulfilling response (confabulated, non-related, "don't know"); and (4) other types of reactions (nil-reactions, echolalic reactions, check-backs, and metacommunicative utterances). This article did not come to my attention until after I had devised my response categories.

   Types of responses which I included in my analysis which I cannot place with certainty within Blanken *et al*'s model are grammatically mismatched responses, question type mismatch, and unmarked topic shifts (although these may be included as examples of "partly fulfilling responses").

as to whether or not the conditions for communication have been satisfied." According to this definition, response slots can be filled not only with answers to questions, but also with requests for clarification (see Garvey 1977, 1979), topic changes, silence, etc.

If the utterance in the response slot is a request for clarification, then any utterance following the answer to the clarification question which is directed to the initial question is counted as a response as well. This situation is illustrated in example 1, in which I ask Elsie about an object on her chest of drawers. After she makes certain that she has correctly identified the object I am asking about (*This one?*), she responds to my original question.

Example 1

HEIDI: Where did you get this?
ELSIE: This one?
HEIDI: Uhhuh.
ELSIE: Oh:: I had it before we were starting and that was kind of a long time ago.

((9) September 5, 1982)

In this case, my question, *Where did you get this?*, is analyzed as having two responses: (1) *This one?* and (2) *Oh:: I had it before we were starting and that was kind of a long time ago.* For the sake of completeness, it should be noted that Elsie's question, *This one?* is analyzed as having one response: *Uhhuh*. Elsie's utterance, *This one?* counts, therefore, both as a question and a response in the overall investigation. The fact that some questions have two responses accounts for the fact that the total number of questions in the analysis to follow is somewhat smaller than the total number of responses.

Each of Elsie's utterances in the response slot following my questions of her was examined according to the following criteria, and determined to be (1) an appropriate response, (2) a vague response, (3) a grammatically mismatched response, (4) a question type mismatch, or (5) no response, as depicted in figure 1 (see p. 115). The identification of utterances in the response slot as being examples of these types is meant to help in tracking the inappropriateness of response which accompanies the progression of Alzheimer's disease. These types are not understood to be in a hierarchical relationship with each other regarding degree of appropriateness. I believe it is premature to make statements to the effect that an unmarked topic shift in the response slot, for example, is somehow more inappropriate than an affirmative answer to a wh-question. Rather, the types of responses seem to be of different *orders*.

Utterances in the response slot were evaluated according to the following criteria:

No response: Did Elsie respond to the question? If Elsie (1) simply continued on with an earlier topic, disregarding the question; (2) introduced a new topic, disregarding the question; or (3) gave no verbal or nonverbal reaction to the question whatsoever (with the usual consequence that I repeated or reformulated the original question following a pause), her utterance following my question was determined to be an example of *no response*. If she gave a response (even if that response was in the form of another question), I went on to the next criterion.

In example 2, Elsie asks me a question in line 1 that I am unable to understand. My request for clarification in line 2 is followed by a 2.2 second silence before I reformulate my question in line 3.

Example 2

1. ELSIE: Will you keep will you keep (till it) please? (0.7)
2. HEIDI: What would you like me to do? (2.2)
3. HEIDI: Will I what?

((12) July 4, 1985)

This 2.2 second silence between my utterances is considered to be *no response* on Elsie's part.

Question type mismatch: Was Elsie apparently able or unable to distinguish between yes–no questions and wh-questions? If the response did not match the type of question asked, e.g. if Elsie responded *yes* to *what's your husband's name?*, it was determined to be an example of *question type mismatch*. If the answer matched the type of question asked (regardless of content), I went on to the next criterion. In the conversation which contains example 3, Elsie is showing me some pictures of tools in a catalogue.

Example 3

HEIDI: What are they used for?
ELSIE: Yes, that's right.

((11) March 17, 1984)

Appropriate response: Was Elsie's response appropriate? This criterion is necessarily somewhat subjective and will differ according to the function of the question (see chapter 3). For example, if the question requests information, does the response provide that information? Here it is important to point out that, since only 4% (15 of 343) of my questions to Elsie were of the "tutorial" type where I knew the answer to the question I was asking, the actual *correctness* of the information provided by Elsie in her responses cannot be evaluated. We are only concerned here with determining whether Elsie provided information which *could* be correct.

In example 4, Elsie has just pointed up into the sky and asked me *Did you see it?*

Example 4

HEIDI: Was there an airplane?
ELSIE: Yes. It was up going up . . there.

((6) March 5, 1982)

Her response to my clarification request "Was there an airplane?" is completely appropriate, although, as noted above, we do not know for a fact that there was indeed an airplane in the sky at that time.

Additionally, the reader may recall the discussion of Yadugiri (1986) in chapters 2 and 3 who argues that a simple answer of *yes* to those yes–no questions which could be meant as indirect wh-questions is "pragmatically inadequate" (e.g. *Did you ever live in someplace like India . . or uh Japan?*). Since speaker intention is difficult to ascertain, however, all of Elsie's simple answers of *yes* to yes–no questions are counted as appropriate answers in this analysis, even though some of them might arguably be seen as pragmatically inappropriate.

If the question requests an action, is that action carried out or challenged? In example 5, I am trying to get Elsie to sit up straighter so that she can drink the water that she has asked for without spilling it.

Example 5

HEIDI: Can you sit up a little more?
ELSIE: Sure. Uhhuh.

((13) July 12, 1985)

Although Elsie provides a verbal response here in addition to her nonverbal action of sitting up, a nonverbal response alone would have also been appropriate.

In addition, as discussed above, it is important to note that an appropriate response to a question need not necessarily be an answer to that question. It is often another question – a signal of acoustic difficulty; a request for additional information necessary to providing an answer to the original question; or a reformulation of the question, often preceded by *you mean ...?* In example 6, Elsie requests additional information (*what time? when?*) before answering my original question about going to exercise class. This is a fully appropriate response.

Example 6

HEIDI: Hi. Would you like to go to exercise class today?
ELSIE: What time? When?

((5) November 27, 1981)

In sum, if the utterance in the response slot was deemed to be "unnoticeably" appropriate, it was determined to be an example of an *appropriate response*. If it seemed unusual, I went on to the next criterion.

Vague response or grammatical mismatch: Was Elsie's response inappropriate because it was vague or because it was mismatched grammatically with the question which elicited it? To clarify this distinction, it will be useful to list several features of responses which led to the decision differentiating these two groups. *Vague responses* (example 7) often contain neologisms or so-called "empty" words, such as *thing*, *place*, and *part*. This vagueness contributes to inappropriateness of the response because the information requested in the question is too nonspecific to be of use to the questioner. *Grammatically mismatched responses* (examples 8 and 9) contain grammatical disagreement (such as pronoun selection, tense, number, or mood). As noted above, the "correctness" of the response is not judged by its match with "real-world" facts.

In example 7, Elsie and I are looking at some porcelain angels in her room. The inappropriateness of Elsie's response to my question about who had given them to her can be traced to its vagueness.

Example 7

HEIDI: Who gave you those?
ELSIE: Well different ones. Some of us.

((9) September 5, 1982)

Table 10. *Appropriateness of Elsie's responses to Heidi's questions in five selected conversations*

(no. = 352)

	appropriate response	vague response	grammatical mismatch	question type mismatch	no response	Totals
3/82	47% (23)	20% (10)	29% (14)	–	4% (2)	49
9/82	64% (34)	17% (9)	15% (8)	2% (1)	2% (1)	53
3/84	39% (26)	11% (7)	18% (12)	18% (12)	14% (9)	66
7/85	45% (51)	9% (10)	2% (2)	4% (4)	39% (43)	110
3/86	51% (38)	–	–	3% (2)	46% (34)	74
Totals	49% (172)	10% (36)	10% (36)	5% (19)	25% (89)	(352)

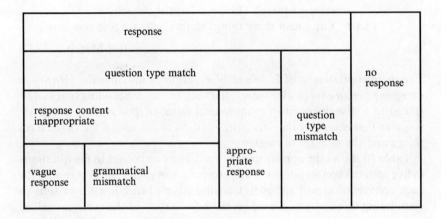

Figure 1. Types of appropriate and inappropriate responses

All that I know from Elsie's answer is that more than one person (*different ones*) gave the angels to her, but have little or no information about their identities (*some of us* could mean "relatives").

In example 8, I was asking Elsie about the previous summer months during which I had not seen her. Her response to a question about the *past* (manifested in the simple past tense form *did* corrected to the present perfect progressive form *have you been going*) in the form of a clarification request containing an adverb referring to a *future* time (*tonight*) is inappropriate.

Example 8

HEIDI: Did uh have you been going to exercise class? or to
cooking class?
ELSIE: Tonight you mean?
HEIDI: With Jill, this summer. ⌐ Did you go?
ELSIE: └ Oh summer. Summer. There
would be.

((9) September 5, 1982)

In example 9, Elsie and I were looking out of the window in the second-
floor lounge.

Example 9

HEIDI: Have you ever gone to that church over there? Across the
street over there? There's a Baptist church.
ELSIE: You mean these things in this little ringlim one here?

((6) March 5, 1982)

The inappropriateness of Elsie's reformulation of my question (*Have you
ever gone to that church over there?*) to check her understanding of it can be
traced to a disagreement in grammatical number (plural *these things* vs.
singular *that church* or *the street*), in addition to her use of the vague term
things and the neologism *ringlim*.

Table 10 shows the appropriateness of Elsie's responses to my questions
in five selected conversations. The percentages of each type of response for
each conversation will aid us in tracking Elsie's breakdown over time in
responding to questions. Based on the information in the table, as well as
on correlations between type of response and fetures of the eliciting
question, several observations can be made.

Discussion of findings

Qualitative changes over time

An examination of the various types of inappropriate responses evidenced
in table 10 points to the fact that Elsie's breakdown in ability to respond
changes *qualitatively* rather than *quantitatively* over time. For example, we
note Elsie's *decreasing* tendency to provide vague responses over time, as
well as a similar trend for responses which disagree grammatically with the
question. Regarding the inappropriateness of a yes–no answer to a wh-
question, we note the relatively high percentage (18%) of such responses

by Elsie in March 1984. The proportion of "no response" increases over time, reaching markedly high numbers in July 1985 (39%) and March 1986 (46%).[2]

Following this hypothesis that the breakdown in appropriateness of response is a *qualitative* and not a quantitative one, we note that in the early conversations the inappropriateness is relatively due to content-level infelicities (either vague or grammatically mismatched) than to structural infelicities (question type mismatch) or the readiness to respond. In other words, in the two early conversations Elsie generally appears to know (1) that she should respond to a question (only 4% and 2% of questions are not responded to), and (2) that the response should match the question type (only one question type mismatch occurs in these two conversations).

Then, a qualitative shift takes place as evidenced in the March 1984 conversation, in which Elsie significantly increases her question type mismatches as well as her "no responses." These sources of inappropriateness join the content-level infelicities characteristic of the first two conversations, which continue to plague this third conversation, to result in the most even distribution of inappropriate responses according to type among the five conversations. Yet another qualitative shift takes place as evidenced in the final two conversations, in which the content-level inappropriate responses play a much smaller role than in the first three conversations, the question type mismatches have dropped back to the relatively insignificant level of the first two conversations, and the proportion of "no responses" increases dramatically.

It has already been observed in the profile of her language use that Elsie's awareness of structure appears to be more complete than her awareness of content (see chapter 2). This differential awareness seems to be at the heart of this breakdown sequence. That the recipient of an utterance needs "to show that he has received the message and correctly" is considered by Goffman (1981: 12) to be one of the "very fundamental requirements of talk as a communication system." This structural condition which entails that a question can expect an answer says nothing

---

[2] It is interesting to compare these findings with those reported in Blanken, Dittmann, Haas, and Wallesch (1987: 267) based on responses given by ten patients with moderate Alzheimer's disease in a "semi-standardized interview" of 5–10 minutes. They found that 42.8% of these patients' responses were "fulfilling responses." When we add to that percentage the 7.2% of responses which were "check-backs" (incorporated in my framework as an appropriate response), we come up with a total of 50% appropriate responses. The percentage of responses which were seen as "partly fulfilling" was 13.9%. These include what I have termed "vague responses." The percentage of patient responses which were termed "non-related" was 13.9%; the percentage of "nil-reactions" was 2.2%. These two percentages combined at 16.1% seem to be approximately equivalent to what I include under the "no-response" category.

about whether that slot will be filled with a response which is type-matched (with regard to yes–no and wh-questions). It is simply very basic knowledge about how humans interact with each other. Also basic but involving linguistic knowledge is type-matching of questions. More specific knowledge about what comprises an appropriate response involves matching of grammatical categories and meshing the specific kinds and amounts of information needed by the questioner. Elsie possesses these types of knowledge and loses them at varying points over time.

Specific analyses of Elsie's responses to wh-questions and questions requesting repetition yield the following insights. Until fall 1982 Elsie's answers to wh-questions are typified by use of inexplicit, "empty," words. During the spring 1984 conversation it is typical for Elsie to answer wh-questions with *yes*. An examination of the fall 1982 conversations gives us insight into a possible transitional stage between these two types of responses to wh-questions. It appears that the precursor to the yes–no responses to wh-questions is a response directed to a different wh-question than the one actually asked. In example 10, Elsie answers a "time" question (*how long?*) with a response regarding location.

> *Example 10*
>
> HEIDI: How long have you had the flowers?
> ELSIE: The flowers?
> HEIDI: Mhm.
> ELSIE: Oh. They're somewhere around.
>
> ((9) September 5, 1982)

Stubbs (1983: 107) observes that, while the reverse is not true, place adverbials can sometimes substitute for time adverbials, e.g. *When did that happen? At the party.* In example 10, however, the answer to *How long* must be either a period of time, such as *three years, since I left home* or reference to an earlier point in time, such as *my son gave them to me in 1978*. Elsie's utterance, *They're around somewhere*, appears to be a response to the question *Where do you have the flowers?*

In example 11, Elsie answers a *where*-question with a *when* answer in reference to an object on her chest of drawers.

> *Example 11*
>
> HEIDI: Where did you get this?
> ELSIE: This one?
> HEIDI: Uhhuh.

ELSIE: Oh:: I had it <u>before</u> we were starting and that was <u>kind of</u>
a long time ago.

((9) September 5, 1982)

In this example the *where*-question is not necessarily requesting a location,
but could be requesting the source of the object. An appropriate answer
could include the name of a city (*In New York*) or the name of a person
who gave the object to Elsie (*From Helen*). Elsie's reference to a point in
time, *before we were starting*, however, responds to the question *When did
you get this?* but does not provide an answer to my question as I posed it.
In light of Elsie's ability at this point to give accounts, her response to my
question might be an account as to why she cannot remember where she
got the object. This interpretation is perhaps easier to see if the phrase, *I
forget*, is inserted between Elsie's *oh::* and the rest of her response.

Following spring 1984, Elsie's typical response to wh-questions is *no*
response. As we trace the development of Elsie's responses to wh-
questions, we find inexplicit responses followed by responses to the
"wrong" wh-question, followed by responses to the wrong *type* of
question (yes–no question rather than wh-question), followed finally by
no response.

Correlation between types of response and features of eliciting questions

In this section several observations are made regarding the possible
influence of a variety of features of my eliciting questions on Elsie's ability
to respond to those questions. These observations are based on correlations between her types of responses (both appropriate and inappropriate)
and features of my questions.

Type of question As would be expected, Elsie responds more
appropriately to yes–no questions than to wh-questions. Of the total
number of questions which receives a fully appropriate response from
Elsie, 80% (132 of 164) are yes–no questions as compared with the
percentage of yes–no questions overall which is only 69% (236 of 343)
($p < 0.01$). Although it may in fact be easier to understand a yes–no
question than a wh-question, certainly we must consider the role which
production factors play. In terms of division of labor, Elsie must do more
work in answering a wh-question whose proposition is incomplete than a
yes–no question whose proposition must only be agreed or disagreed with.
In light of the word-finding difficulties which accompany Alzheimer's
disease, it is not surprising that it is easier for Elsie to say *yes* or *no* than to
give a more elaborate answer to a wh-question. In fact, she may even

answer *yes* or *no* without understanding the question. In their study of the pragmatic abilities of late-stage Alzheimer's patients Causino, Obler, Knoefel, and Albert (forthcoming) also found that their patients responded more appropriately to yes–no questions than to wh-questions whose responses tended to be "irrelevant, incoherent or absent."

Looking specifically at the content-level inappropriateness of Elsie's responses to wh-questions, which is especially typical of the conversations before 1984, we find that she responds vaguely rather than in a grammatically mismatched way. Of the total number of questions which receive a vague response, 49% (17 of 35) are wh-questions as compared with 17% (60 of 343) representation overall (significant at the 1% level). On the other hand, of the total number of questions which receive a grammatically mismatched response, 17% (6 of 35) are wh-questions as compared with 17% (60 of 343) representation overall. This finding indicates that, in the early conversations at least, Elsie understands the question, in that she uses grammatical categories in her response which match those in the question. The problem in this case appears to be on the production level, in that Elsie lacks the *exact* lexical item(s) to respond and must resort to using "empty" words, neologisms, or circumlocutions.

Influences on lack of response   Although it seems as if it should be easy for Elsie simply to repeat what she just said, responses to questions requesting repetition (*hmm? huh?*) appear to give her the most trouble of all in our conversations. Elsie does not respond to 58% (11 of 19) of all questions which indicate an acoustic problem in comprehension (*huh?, hmm?*). This finding is surprising. Why would Elsie ignore my requests that she repeat an utterance which was not heard well enough to enable the conversation to continue? An examination of Elsie's responses to my requests for repetition (*hmm? huh?*) in spring 1984 through spring 1986 (no clear case of such a question on my part exists in the earlier conversations) reveals similarities to wh-question responses regarding the breakdown sequence. During the conversations of spring 1984 and summer 1985, Elsie responds occasionally, as is the case for wh-questions, with an affirmative answer, such as *yes* or *mhm*.

Example 12 shows one instance of Elsie giving an affirmative answer to a request for repetition. While I am showing her a brightly colored feather, Elsie says something I do not understand and I ask her to repeat it. When she does not repeat what she said earlier, I tell her that I did not hear her before, to which she says something else I do not understand. In response to my *hmm?*, Elsie responds in the affirmative (*Yes. Oh yes. Sure*) and continues my talk about the feather by reformulating what I had said in the first line of the example (*so many color*).

Example 12

HEIDI: All sorts of colors. Almost matches your . . dress.
ELSIE: [clears throat] and then seven(teen) . . (to dear) honey.
HEIDI: What? What did you just say?
ELSIE: (hmm)
HEIDI: I didn't hear you.
ELSIE: Oh let's see. (which which which?) ()
HEIDI: <u>Hmm?</u>
ELSIE: <u>Yes. Oh yes. Sure.</u> So many so many color.
HEIDI: So many colors? . . . . .

((13) July 12, 1985)

It is as if all of the utterances in between were nonexistent. The fact that Elsie is able to maintain a topic by reformulating my utterance should not cloud Elsie's inability to respond appropriately to my requests for repetition.

This type of response was involved in an interesting "clash" involving Elsie's and my discourse strategies. Due to greater-than-before comprehension problems on my part in the summer 1985 conversations, I had been employing a strategy of listening hard for and jumping on the first recognizable word in Elsie's utterances. I would then incorporate that word into my next turn, usually in the form of a question to check my understanding of what Elsie had just said. In example 13, when I do not understand Elsie's response to my question about whether she would like to drink some more water, I ask for a repetition (*Hmm?*), to which she employs her strategy of responding affirmatively (*I think so*). Upon recognizing the verb *think* in Elsie's utterance, I incorporateit into my next question of her, to which I receive no response from Elsie.

Example 13

HEIDI: Would you like a little more water?
ELSIE: (And you prob). They were (they were) () days (cause
    dear) . . course, dear.
HEIDI: <u>Hmm?</u>
ELSIE: <u>I think so.</u>
HEIDI: <u>What do you think?</u> . . . . .

((13) July 12, 1985)

In spring 1986, Elsie gives no response to my requests for repetition. Example 14 illustrates how this phenomenon looks in a conversation in which Elsie uses only tokens of *uhhuh, mhm, mm Hm, mmm* and *hmm?*.

> *Example 14*
>
> HEIDI: I'll show ⌐ you
> ELSIE: ⌐ mhm ⌐
> HEIDI: └ Hmm? (15.8) Here I'll show you a
> picture.
>
>   ((14) March 18, 1986)

In this example, I break off my utterance to respond immediately to Elsie's utterance which overlapped with mine. Because of the overlap, I did not hear what Elsie had said, only that she had said something. I need her to repeat (and possibly elaborate on) what she has just said. But Elsie does not respond, and after waiting 15.8 seconds, I continue with my original utterance. It is not possible to determine here whether Elsie does not understand the purpose of repeating what she just said or whether she does not understand the request made of her.

It is interesting, on the other hand, to note that Elsie herself uses this type of question (seemingly) to request repetition in March 1986; it seems unlikely that she could not comprehend a type of question that she can produce appropriately, but the apparent paradox may be accounted for by the notion of automaticity. It may be that Elsie is using *hmm?* automatically in the later conversations without necessarily knowing what its function is.[3]

Both in Elsie's responses to wh-questions and to requests for repetition, it does not appear that there is any advantage to one type of inappropriate response over another with regard to comprehension by the conversational partner. They all seem to lead astray. The change in type of response seems, rather, to be related to the relative amount of effort needed to produce a response. It is, of course, easiest in terms of linguistic production not to respond at all. If one does respond, it is easier to respond with one word, *yes*, than to produce a longer utterance, either of the inexplicit type or of the misguided type (answer to another wh-question), in the case of wh-questions, or repetition in full of one's earlier utterance in the case of requests for repetition.

Otherwise, there appears to be no relationship between question

---

[3] I am grateful to an anonymous reviewer for the notion that this paradoxical situation may be related to my earlier discussion of the role of automaticity of language in Elsie's communicative behavior.

features and Elsie's lack of response. It seems that Elsie more-or-less randomly does not respond to questions. Both wh- and yes–no questions are approximately equally underrepresented in this category. All functions are represented approximately in the same proportion as in my eliciting questions. Temporal reference in the question seems to make no difference. Eighty-four percent (59 of 70) of yes–no questions and wh-questions which receive no response refer to the present time, 13% (9 of 70) refer to the past, and 3% (2 of 70) refer to the future. When these numbers are compared with my temporal reference during the final three conversations when the vast majority of the "no responses" occur (86 of 89), the finding is statistically insignificant. During those three conversations, 88% of my questions (182 of 208) refer to the present time, 11% (24 of 208) refer to the past, and only 1% (2 of 208) refer to the future.

Temporal reference Of the total number of questions which receive an appropriate response from Elsie, 83% (119 of 144) refer to the present time as compared with 79% (235 of 298) overall which refer to the present time. Accordingly, only 16% (25 of 144) of questions which refer to the past or the future receive an appropriate response compared with their representation overall of 21% (62 of 298). These findings are not statistically significant and indicate that Elsie is not hindered in her ability to design an appropriate response to questions which refer to the past or to the future, nor is it easier for her to respond appropriately to questions about the present time.

Although this finding that the temporal reference of a question does not seem to help or hinder Elsie in the production of an appropriate response comes as somewhat of a surprise, we find a more expected situation when we examine the relationship between Elsie's grammatically mismatched responses and the temporal reference of the eliciting question. Elsie does tend to give a response which disagrees grammatically with the question to yes–no questions which request information about times other than the present. Forty-nine percent (17 of 35) of grammatically mismatched responses are to questions which refer to times other than the present; this number contrasts with 21% (62 of 298) representation of questions with reference to times other than the present overall (this finding is statistically significant at the 1% level). Further analyses indicate that a question's temporal reference is more decisive than either the grammatical type or the function of question in eliciting a response which is grammatically mismatched with the question.

Spatial reference Of Elsie's total number of appropriate responses, 87% (125 of 144) are to yes–no questions, wh-questions, and alternative questions whose spatial reference is proximal and 13% (19 of 144) are to those questions whose spatial reference is distal. This is in exact agreement with the overall proportions in my eliciting questions. Out of 298 yes–no questions, wh-questions, and alternative questions asked, 259 have proximal reference (87%). This finding indicates strongly that the spatial reference of my questions neither helps nor hinders Elsie in her responses to these questions.

Accommodation to perceived abilities

As we track the breakdown in Elsie's ability to respond to questions, we must also take into account the general decline in her health, including loss of energy and initiative, which may result in a lower level of creative language production and of the ability to take the perspective of the conversational partner into account. This situation is then coupled with my own (unintentional) accommodation to my perceptions of Elsie's declining abilities along the way, which buoys the interaction up, allowing Elsie to look more successful as a conversational partner than she actually is.

This accommodation on my part to Elsie's decreasing abilities to answer questions accounts for the otherwise puzzling fact that Elsie's percentage of appropriate responses does not decrease steadily along with the progression of the disease. The highest percentage of appropriate responses made by Elsie occurred in September 1982 (63% of total responses). The lowest percentage occurred in March 1984 (39%), with 51% of Elsie's responses in March 1986 being interpreted as appropriate. Upon closer examination of the data, it appears that in selecting the *type* of question to ask her, I was attuning to my preconceptions of Elsie's ability to answer various types of questions. This strategy enabled Elsie *despite decreasing abilities* to continue to give a high proportion of appropriate responses. In March 1984, when Elsie had the lowest percentage of appropriate responses of the five conversations (39%), I asked the greatest number of wh-questions (39%) and the smallest number of yes–no questions (52%) of all five conversations. Keeping this in mind, it comes as no surprise that Elsie's proportion of appropriate responses actually *increases* in the July 1985 (45%) and March 1986 (51%) conversations, when I used a decreasing number of wh-questions (8% in July 1985 and 8% in March 1986) and an increasing number of yes–no questions (69% in July 1985 and 78% in March 1986). In adjusting my questioning strategies to match what I perceived to be Elsie's decreasing ability to provide appropriate responses to wh-questions, I not only attuned to Elsie's ability to comprehend but also allowed Elsie's next move to be an appropriate one.

Example 15 illustrates how this accommodation of question type can take place within a very short time span, as the listener's inability to deal with the more difficult question types becomes apparent to the speaker. The example begins with Elsie asking me a question in lines 1–2 which I am unable to understand. As the conversation progresses, Elsie's actions indicate that she wants me to push away the protective railing which runs along the side of her bed.

Example 15

1. ELSIE: Will you keep will you keep (till it)
2. please? (0.7)
3. HEIDI: <u>What would you like me to do?</u> (2.2)
4. <u>Will I what?</u> (3.5)
5. ELSIE: And they (get uh get themselves) to
6. push this (here. I didn't, here.
7. right) (0.4)
8. HEIDI: <u>What would you like to be pushed?</u>
9. (0.3) <u>This?</u>

((12) July 4, 1985)

The accommodation begins with my reformulation of an unmarked open-ended wh-question (*What would you like me to do?*) into a marked open-ended wh-question (*Will I what?*) when the unmarked version receives no response (2.2 second pause). This marked form which echoes the syntactic structure of Elsie's question can be seen as an attempt to ease Elsie's next turn, the reproduction of her original question. Following a somewhat confusing utterance 3.5 seconds after the marked open-ended question (lines 5, 6, and 7), which, contrary to my expectations, is not posed within the *will X . .?* framework, I incorporate the verb Elsie's response contained (*push*) into an unmarked, but focused, wh-question (*What would you like to be pushed?*). I then immediately continue with a focused yes–no question (*This?*), pointing to the railing on the side of her bed. This question asks only for confirmation of its content by Elsie, allowing her to do an even smaller share of the discourse work. Thus, the sequence clearly shows the continual adjustments made in question formation to accommodate Elsie's apparent inability to comprehend my question with the intent to facilitate her next conversational move. This question sequence is typical of Elsie's and my exchanges in the later conversations of 1985 and 1986, as Elsie becomes less able to do discourse work.

Production as a key to comprehension level

In the later stages of Alzheimer's disease, when the patient has a very limited communicative repertoire, it is often difficult to ascertain the level of the patient's comprehension. In their study of end-stage Alzheimer's disease, Causino, Obler, Knoefel, and Albert (forthcoming) focus primarily on the patients' production behaviors, but they call for additional study in the "important, yet relatively unexplored" area of receptive pragmatic skills of these patients. In this section, I examine Elsie's questions and responses in our conversation of March 1986 to provide evidence that even Elsie's extremely limited linguistic production at an advanced stage of the disease can be used as a key to her level of comprehension. The apparent systematicity of Elsie's use of *hmm?, mhm, mm Hm,* and *mmm* (which only became clear to me during microanalysis following the conversation) indicates that Elsie's level of comprehension is indeed higher than her production problems allow her to show in an ongoing conversation.

In our conversation on March 18, 1986, Elsie asks a total of three questions, all *hmm?,* and all in response to a yes–no question including the word *you.* Following Elsie's *hmm?* each of the above questions is repeated immediately and exactly. The balance of Elsie's linguistic contributions are all responses to my utterances. In other words, Elsie never once initiates an exchange *linguistically* in this conversation. All of her questions and her statements are in response to something I said. This supports findings by Causino *et al.* that the ten end-stage Alzheimer's patients in their study rarely initiated communication, but were primarily in the respondent's role. I emphasize the word *linguistically* in the statement above, because several times Elsie initiates an exchange by her *actions,* in the sense that I respond to something Elsie is doing to keep the conversation moving along. Examples 16 and 17 illustrate this kind of exchange. In example 16, Elsie's chewing motion initiates a topic shift from talk about friends to talk about food, because I *choose* to elaborate on Elsie's actions, placing her in the initiator role.

Example 16

HEIDI: I spent some time with some friends yesterday.
ELSIE: [chewing motion with mouth]
HEIDI: Looks like you're eating something.
ELSIE: Mhm mhm.
HEIDI: [chuckles] I don't think you are though. I don't think there's anything to eat right now.

In example 17 Elsie directs her gaze away from me toward a picture on the wall, during my questions to her about whether or not she needs a Kleenex. I follow Elsie's lead by talking about the picture for a while before I go to get a tissue for her nose.

Example 17

HEIDI: Do you need another Kleenex?

ELSIE: [directs gaze away from Heidi toward picture]

HEIDI: Are you looking at the picture? This one? Isn't that pretty?
Those colors. It says it's by Sally. Do you know Sally? Sally.
Do you know that person? . . . Isn't that pretty? [leaves to get
Kleenex]

With the exception of one token of *uhhuh*, all of Elsie's responses were
of three types: *mhm* (62 tokens), *mm Hm* (9 tokens), and *mmm* (7 tokens).
Whereas *mhm* seems to serve as an "all-purpose" response for Elsie in this
conversation, one which is used to fulfill conditional relevance (and this is
indeed the response used in the inappropriate yes–no responses to wh-
questions), *mm Hm* (same as *mhm* but with greater emphasis on the
second syllable) seems to be a definite affirmative response. Example 18
illustrates Elsie's response to seeing a photograph of herself.

Example 18

HEIDI: [gets a photograph] Look at this one. Do you know this
person?

ELSIE: Mhm. ⌐ Mhm.

HEIDI: ⌐ [chuckles] That's you!

ELSIE: Mm Hm.

Example 19 occurs after I got Elsie a Kleenex and helped her blow her
nose.

Example 19

HEIDI: Here. Here you go. Is that what you need? Yeah.

ELSIE: [blows nose]

HEIDI: Can you blow hard? Is that better?

ELSIE: Mhm. [clearly said]

HEIDI: Yeah. ⌐ Good. [laughs] That's what you

ELSIE: ⌐ Mhm.

HEIDI: needed.

ELSIE: Mm Hm.

Our biggest indication of Elsie's comprehension level, amid the meager
amount of verbal production, however, is Elsie's use of *mmm*. Of the seven
occurrences of *mmm* in the conversation, six are in response to emotional

utterances or situations for Elsie. Two occurrences are in response to my
showing Elsie a photograph of her family, as illustrated by example 20.

> *Example 20*
> HEIDI: Do you wanna see a picture?
> ELSIE: Mhm.
> HEIDI: Yeah? I'll see if you know who this is. Just a second. [gets
>   picture of Elsie's husband] Look at this. Who's that?
> ELSIE: Mmmmm. [high to low pitch contour]

Two occurrences are in response to *I love you (Elsie)*, as illustrated by
example 21.

> *Example 21*
> HEIDI: I'll go now. ⌐
> ELSIE: └ Mhm.
> HEIDI: I'm sure glad I got to see you though.
>   I love you. ⌐
> ELSIE: └ Mmmm. Mhm.

One occurrence is in response to *You're a sweet lady* as illustrated by
example 22.

> *Example 22*
> HEIDI: You're a sweet lady [chuckles]
> ELSIE: Mmm. ⌐ [chuckles]
> HEIDI: └ You are a sweet lady. ⌐
> ELSIE: └ Mhm mmm.

One occurrence is in response to *I'm glad you're still here, so that I could
find you.* The only *mmm* used by Elsie to a somewhat less personally
emotional topic is when I show her some *National Geographic* magazines,
which she used to love to read. Bartol's observation (1982 as cited in
Causino, Obler, Knoefel, and Albert, forthcoming) that individuals with
advanced Alzheimer's disease are highly sensitive to such paralinguistic
aspects of communication as rate, loudness, pitch, and intonation, *especially as these are used to convey emotion or affect* (as opposed to the
communication of propositional meaning) suggests that Elsie may be
responding as much to (or even more than) the emotional paralinguistic
aspects of what I said than to its actual emotional semantic content.

Another clue to Elsie's ability to comprehend is provided by example 16 above. Elsie's chewing motion in the absence of food makes a good deal more sense when we note that three turns earlier I asked Elsie *Did you have your lunch yet?* Since this is the only time in the conversation that I talk about food and Elsie's chewing motion only occurs this one time during the conversation, it seems likely that Elsie indeed (at some level) comprehends the meaning of the word *lunch*.

In sum, the limited linguistic means used by Elsie in the conversation of March 1986 gives us insights into her level of comprehension. Exploring beyond the seemingly indiscriminate and overwhelming use of *mhm* (78% of responses vs. 9% *mmm*, 11% *mm Hm*, and 1% *uhhuh*), we note that Elsie apparently is able (1) to determine when she needs a question to be repeated in order to give it an answer (her use of *hmm?*), (2) to distinguish between emotional topics (*mmm*) and more banal ones (*mhm*), and (3) to make the link between the semantic meaning of selected lexical items apart from their physical context and appropriate related activities (*lunch* and chewing action). It is important here to point to parallel findings that aphasic patients seem to respond better to emotional topics (Andresen 1986) and an observation by Sabat, Wiggs, and Pinizzotto (1984) during home visits to Alzheimer's patients that these patients often can respond appropriately to potential crisis or danger situations, such as a child venturing too near a hot stove.

In closing the discussion of Elsie's responses to my questions, it is interesting to note the ways in which the qualitative changes in appropriateness of response to questions interact with two other types of changes in the discourse to create a more complete characterization of the three quantitatively different stages of discourse production discussed above. Table 2 (see page 90) indicates the relative amount of verbal participation of the two interlocutors in each conversation by a simple count of words uttered. Here we note that Elsie's proportion of talk (69%–80%) remains substantially higher than that of her partner (20%–31%) in the first three conversations, dropping to 28% and 12% in the final two conversations.

Table 1 (see page 89) indicates the proportion of questions asked by both interlocutors in each conversation. Here we note that Elsie's proportion of questions asked remains higher (57%) than that of her partner in the first two conversations, drops off somewhat (37%) in the third conversation, and falls to the low levels of 7% and 4% in the final two conversations.

Combining the information on Elsie's relative degree of participation in these five conversations, as gleaned from tables 1 and 2, with the information regarding her appropriateness of response as discussed above, we can provide the following characterizations of three qualitatively different stages in the patient's discourse production.

Stage 1 is characterized by (1) a high percentage of content-level inappropriate responses relative to structural-level inappropriate responses; (2) a high level of patient participation in conversation in terms of percentage of total number of words produced; and (3) a high level of patient participation in conversation in terms of percentage of total number of questions asked.

Stage 2 is characterized by (1) relatively even distribution of all types of inappropriate responses (content-level inappropriateness somewhat lower than in stage 1; structural-level inappropriateness somewhat higher than in stage 1); (2) continued high level of patient participation in conversation in terms of percentage of total number of words produced; and (3) somewhat lower patient participation in conversation in terms of percentage of total number of questions asked than in stage 1.

Stage 3 is characterized by (1) virtually no content-level inappropriateness of response. Inappropriateness of response is largely due to "no response" (silence, change of topic, continuation of earlier topic); (2) substantially reduced level of patient participation in conversation in terms of percentage of total number of words produced than in stages 1 and 2; and (3) significantly lower patient participation in conversation in terms of percentage of total number of questions asked than in stages 1 and 2.

Response as discourse strategy

In the sections above we traced the path of Elsie's communication breakdown in terms of her responses to questions over time. In this section we examine *my* responses to *Elsie's* questions, applying the same appropriateness criteria which were developed for use with *Elsie's* responses to *my* questions. According to these criteria, a small number of my responses are judged to be inappropriate. Reexamination indicates that attention to face issues in the interaction may have motivated the "inappropriate" response design. A tridimensional model (figure 2: see page 133) is then presented in which responses are placed according to the relative amount of speaker focus on the interactional goals of coherence, positive face maintenance, and negative face maintenance. Against this backdrop Elsie's responses, judged to be inappropriate earlier in this chapter, are reexamined to determine whether face concerns rather than communicative disability may have resulted in their design. There it is suggested that the lack of possible motivation for face concerns in Elsie's inappropriate utterances generally justify different interpretations of similar response strategies used by Elsie and me.

Table 11. *Appropriateness ratings of Heidi's responses in five selected conversations*

	appropriate response	vague response	grammatical mismatch	question type mismatch	no response
3/82	88% (53)	–	7% (4)	–	5% (3)
9/82	85% (57)	–	4% (3)	–	9% (6)
3/84	74% (29)	–	–	5% (2)	21% (8)
7/85	75% (6)	–	–	–	25% (2)
3/86	100% (3)	–	–	–	–

Interactional goals as determinants of response strategy

As table 11 indicates, a small percentage of my responses were judged to be inappropriate when the appropriateness criteria developed for use with Elsie's responses were applied to my responses. Upon closer examination of my responses to Elsie's questions, the inappropriate responses tend to fall into four basic groups:
(1) a response which disagrees grammatically with Elsie's question which elicited it;
(2) a response which does not match the type of Elsie's eliciting question;
(3) no response to Elsie's question (pause, continuation of old topic, or initiation of new topic);
(4) a response which is, by definition, appropriate in the sense that it matches the question type, agrees grammatically with the question that elicited it, and is not vague. However, because of a mismatch between Elsie's question design and reality, and the resultant problems in understanding on my part, my response, though technically appropriate, is somehow odd.

I suggest that what these various types of inappropriate or odd responses have in common is that they are produced in the face of communicative breakdown. Such responses appear to be produced as a result of a comprehension problem either on Elsie's or my part.

Following Lakoff's (1973, 1979) discussion of clarity and politeness in conversation, utterance design in response to a communicative breakdown can be seen as negotiative between coherence and face-maintenance. "Face" is defined by Goffman (1967: 5) as "the positive social value a person effectively claims for himself by the line others assume he has taken during a particular contact. Face is an image of self delineated in terms of approved social attributes." Lakoff (1973) maintains that in most informal conversations face issues are more important than clarity, because "actual communication of important ideas is secondary to merely reaffirming and strengthening relationships." Reacting to what she believed to be undue emphasis on information transfer by Grice (1975) in his discussion of the Cooperative Principle and its maxims, Lakoff (1973) introduces a rule-based analysis of politeness. These rules, which Lakoff calls *Rules of Politeness* (1. don't impose; 2. give options; 3. be friendly) are presented as a way to determine which of the corresponding notions of distance, deference, and camaraderie are most characteristic of a person's overall communicative style. Tannen's (1984) subsequent discussion of conversational style focuses on the relative value an individual places on involvement and independence. That is, all of us fluctuate between our need for individuality and our need for belonging to a group, and this fluctuation is reflected in our language use. Our conversational style is determined along the continuum running between involvement and independence, depending on which of the two is more important to us.

Tannen's discussion of involvement and independence points essentially to the same two conflicting human needs as represented by the terms *positive* and *negative face* in Brown and Levinson (1978, 1987). Negative politeness is that which anoints a person's negative face, i.e. takes into account the interlocutor's need for independence. Positive politeness is that which anoints a person's positive face, i.e. takes into account his or her need to be liked and to have his or her wishes understood. However, while Lakoff's and Tannen's goals are a systematic way to discuss communicative and conversational style, respectively, Brown and Levinson's primary goal is strategic determination of the linguistic manifestations of the two types of politeness.

I would like to suggest that the interactional goals of coherence,[4] positive face maintenance, and negative face maintenance be seen as three axes defining a tridimensional space within which response strategies can be placed. My claim here is not that particular strategies can be distinguished quantitatively from one another by exact placement within the space, rather that they can be compared to one another regarding relative focus on the three goals.

Response strategies aimed at reversing the *linguistic* consequence of communicative breakdown, incoherence, would have coherence as their goal; strategies aiming at reversing one of the *social* consequences of

---

[4] Here I am using the term "coherence" to refer to the clear connections between ideas, actions, or both, in discourse. This is to be differentiated from cohesion, as discussed by Halliday and Hasan (1976), which refers to linguistic connections on the surface level of spoken utterances or written sentences. It is also a somewhat more narrow interpretation of coherence than that made by Schiffrin (1987), as discussed in chapter 1 of the present study.

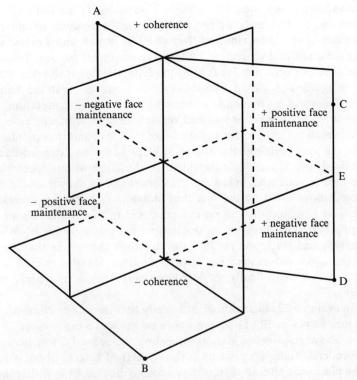

Figure 2. Tridimensional response strategy space

communicative breakdown, a feeling of helplessness and dependence, would have negative face maintenance as their goal; and finally, strategies aimed at reversing another *social* consequence of communicative break-down, a feeling of being an undesirable person, would have positive face maintenance as their goal.

In what follows, I discuss strategies used to respond to communicative breakdowns in interactions involving Elsie and me with reference to figure 2. The dichotomy of strategies for dealing with face problems discussed by Goffman (1967), *corrective* and *avoidance* strategies, serves as the basic framework for this discussion. However, this framework is expanded to accommodate other hybrid strategies which attempt partial accomplishment of the goals of coherence, positive face maintenance, and negative face maintenance.

   Correction   First, if I perceive understanding to be more important than face issues in the interaction, I can take actions to *correct* a misunderstanding inherent in *Elsie's* question. Other-initiated repairs, however, conflict with the preference for self-correction in conversation (see Schegloff, Jefferson, and Sacks 1977). Brown and Levinson (1987: 38) maintain that correction by the conversational partner threatens the mistaken person's positive face by implying that he or she is incompetent or misguided. I would like to suggest, however, that the context of disabled speakers demands a somewhat different interpretation. Within this context, such other-initiated repair seems to represent an equal (or even greater) threat to the negative face, to the extent that pointing out a mistake may highlight the degree of helplessness and dependence of the disabled individual, while the threat to the disabled interlocutor's positive face is somewhat offset by the consideration shown to the positive face demonstrated by the fact that individual's question is answered at all. This heightened focus on independence in this context seems to find support in the discussion of doctor–patient relationships by Wiemann, Gravell, and Wiemann (1990: 230), in which they argue that the ability to maintain self-control is "always an issue for the elderly, who are seen (either realistically or stereotypically) as in a general state of decline."[5]

In example 23, Elsie thinks incorrectly that the current time of day is 2 o'clock (it is actually 11:30 a.m.) because she sees a big wooden '2' on the wall above the nurses' station indicating the second floor. Because this misunderstanding occurs within the context of talking about a party to take place that afternoon, it is important to me that Elsie realize the party will begin at 2 o'clock, not that it is 2 o'clock now.

Example 23

ELSIE: Well this is nu two now, isn't it? ⌐
HEIDI: └ Yes.
        No. No. No. It's only about 11:30 now.

((3) November 20, 1981)

Following my initial *yes* to her question, either influenced by her use of a negative tag question or by my thinking that she was referring to her floor

---

5   Baltes (1991) notes a disparity between staff and patient perceptions of independence and dependence within institutions for the elderly. She finds that, while staff attribute a patient's dependence to that patient's personality, elderly patients tend to attribute dependence to illness or staff behavior. Regarding the independence of a patient, she finds that staff tend to attribute this independence to efforts made by staff; elderly patients, on the other hand, attribute independence to their own abilities (cf. also Pincus 1981, chapter 4, for a discussion of the relative needs for independence/dependence in old age).

number, I corrected her explicitly by using three *no*'s and following with the correct time.

Additionally, I can use a corrective strategy to attempt to remedy a comprehension problem on *my* part, for example, by asking for further clarification or by stating that I do not understand. In example 24, Elsie uses the personal pronoun *she* with no referent in the physical environment nor in the prior discourse.

Example 24

> ELSIE: She was around yesterday, wasn't she? When they were go
> .. walking around, talking with the groups here?
> HEIDI: Mm. Which one?
> ELSIE: Well it's not she's one of them that has the pretty uh she
> fixes a pretty tray too.

((6) March 5, 1982)

Since I cannot possibly know who *she* refers to, I ask for further clarification, which Elsie attempts to give. Although she cannot supply a proper name, she does provide a clue that *she* is on the staff by telling me that *she fixes a pretty tray* (probable reference to the trays on which meals are served at the health care center).

The approximate location within figure 2 of these examples of corrective strategy is represented by point A, which takes into account the emphasis on coherence, the threat to negative face and the somewhat offsetting consequences with regard to positive face.

Avoidance   Second, if I perceive face issues to be more important than understanding of a proposition in the situation, I can *avoid* talking about Elsie's misunderstanding. Specifically, I can choose for *interactional* reasons not to fulfill her structural discourse expectations, e.g. blatantly not answer Elsie's question. Brown and Levinson (1987: 34) suggest that the choice not to answer can be perceived as a threat to the mistaken person's positive face, in that nonanswers may imply lack of consideration because they show that the interlocutors are not "cooperatively involved in the relevant activity" (1987: 125). This strategy carries with it face-threatening consequences for the person carrying out the act as well, in that he or she has been shown to be uncooperative or inept in terms of the sequential necessities of conversations. Because the avoidance strategy by definition avoids direct reference to the source of the misunderstanding, it also avoids threatening the mistaken person's negative face. Sacrificing the disabled partner's positive face to save her negative face points to an underlying assumption that feelings of independence are relatively more important in this case than feelings of being liked. In example 25, the staff member and I appear to be accommodating to a preconception regarding strong desires on the part of elderly individuals to be independent, as discussed above.

The precontext to example 25, which occurs after example 23 above, involved continued confusion on Elsie's part regarding when and where the party would be that afternoon. My reminding Elsie that she lives on the second floor prompts her to conclude incorrectly that the party will be on the second floor. When Elsie does not relent in asking if her understanding of the situation is correct (it is not), a staff member and I avoid answering her question, choosing instead to change the topic of conversation from the upcoming party to the lunch Elsie is about to eat. (I understand Elsie's use of the word *side* to refer to the wing of the building.)

Example 25

ELSIE: Is that right? (on) which side will it? on which on which side will will it be?
STAFF: You have a good lunch. ⌐
HEIDI: ⌐ Have a good lunch.

((3) November 20, 1981)

Additionally, I can use an avoidance strategy in response to a comprehension problem on *my* part, if I perceive mutual face in the interaction to be more important than my understanding of what is going on. In the interaction containing example 26, Elsie and I are looking at an order blank from a mail-order catalogue. Elsie asks me the following question (*Can uh you put some of your perries?*) which I do not understand and did not answer, despite Elsie's repeated attempts (*dear, dear honey? Lovin? Honey dear? Honey?*) to get my attention. She appears finally to give up hope of getting a response and continues her turn-at-talk.

Example 26

ELSIE: Now are you? (0.4) Can uh you put some of your (perries), dear, dear honey? (0.6) Lovin'? (0.9) Honey dear? (0.8) Honey dear? (1.2) (You well some of it was the re: uh rest.) Yeah.
HEIDI: Uhhuh.
ELSIE: (Did they do any on you righ) yours too? (well then) you put it on

((11) March 17, 1984)

In example 27, after Elsie starts eating her dinner, I say goodbye and start to leave. Then with what I perceive to be a command (*Come back (for sister)*), Elsie initiates a round of utterances which I find confusing. I try to clear up my confusion by asking *Excuse me?*, *What'd you say?*, and the more focused question *Come back for what?* Despite a possible attempt to clarify by another resident (*They seem to be in your ((fat))*) and a double appeal by Elsie (*Wait a minute. Wait a minute*), when Elsie asks a question of her own (*Which is it gonna be?*) at the end of that round, I am so confused that I just say goodbye and leave.

Example 27

HEIDI: Enjoy your dinner.
ELSIE: Thank you.
HEIDI: Bye-bye.
ELSIE: <u>Come back</u> (for sister)
HEIDI: <u>Excuse me?</u>
ELSIE: (They) look (better) anyway.
HEIDI: <u>What'd you say?</u>
ELSIE: They (cleb) anyway.
HEIDI: <u>Come back for what?</u>
ELSIE: (I think for the be)
RESIDENT: They seem to be in your (fat).
ELSIE: Wait a minute. Wait a minute. <u>Which is</u>
    <u>it gonna be?</u> ⌐ It's going to be right
HEIDI: ∟ Right. Okay. Bye-bye.
ELSIE: there. Now wait a minute. <u>Is it gonna</u>
    <u>be? It that gonna be (down in there)?</u>

((11) March 17, 1984)

The approximate location in figure 2 of these examples of avoidance strategy is represented by point B, which takes into account the relative emphasis on negative face and the negative effects on positive face and coherence which would have been facilitated by a suitable response to Elsie's question.

In their study of the communicative competence of another cognitively disabled group, the severely mentally retarded, Price-Williams and Sabsay (1979: 47) point out that this type of avoidance of direct reference to the source of the communicative breakdowns may not be as benevolent to the mentally disabled as it at first appears. They argue that the distress in conversations between retarded and nonretarded interlocutors is at least partially attributable to the failure on the part of the nonretarded individual to report his or her comprehension difficulties to the retarded speaker.

Hybrid strategies   Third, if I do not wish to point directly to Elsie's misunderstanding by using *no* or some similar linguistic feature, but I do want to get across the correct information, I can change the relevant lexical item or grammatical category which is incorrect in my partner's utterance in the design of my own next utterance. In example 28, after I tell Elsie I cannot stay to look at her magazine because I am planning to go downtown with some friends who have arrived from New York, she responds with a tag question (*He's gonna be here for a while then, isn't he?*). Her question includes the personal pronoun *he* which triggers the disagreement in number (plural vs. singular) in my response (*M: my friends will just be here until tomorrow morning. So they won't be here too long*) to her question. Note the elongation of the *m* in *my* in line 15 which may be due to hesitation caused by my having to design a grammatical disagreement. Elsie's incorporation of my change in number into her next turn in lines 20–21 (*So they'll get together and go, won't they?*) indicates the success of this strategy.

Example 28

```
 1. HEIDI: I think I'll have to come back another
 2.        time to look at those ┌ because I'm I'm
 3. ELSIE:                        └ yes
 4. HEIDI: waiting. I have some friends from out
 5.        of town who are here now . .┌ in from New
 6. ELSIE:                             └ mhm
 7. HEIDI: York. So ┌ I'm going ┌ downtown with
 8. ELSIE:          └ Goo:d.     └ Goo:d.
 9. HEIDI: them. ┌ But I wanted to stop by and
10. ELSIE:       └ oh that's fine
11. HEIDI: see you first.
12. ELSIE: Uhhuh. Good. Good. ┌ He's gonna be here
13. HEIDI:                     └ uhhuh.
14. ELSIE: for a while then, isn't he?
15. HEIDI: M: my friends will just be here until
16.        tomorrow morning. ┐
17. ELSIE:                    └ uhhuh ┐
18. HEIDI:                            └ so they
19.        won't be here too long.
20. ELSIE: Oh I see. So they'll get together
21.        and ┌ go, won't they? ┐
22. HEIDI:     └ mhm              └ mhm mhm.
```

((9) September 5, 1982)

Example 29 illustrates this phenomenon carried out by placement of a lexical item rather than of a grammatical category. The situation here is the same as in examples 23 and 25 above, i.e., that Elsie is trying to understand what time the party will take place that afternoon at the center.

Example 29

ELSIE: Oh and where .. what time will that .. that be?
STAFF: Around two th .. two o'clock or one thirty.
ELSIE: Two. ⌐ Two in the <u>morning?</u>
HEIDI: └ Yeah.
STAFF: In the <u>afternoon.</u> ⌐
HEIDI: └ Two in the <u>afternoon.</u>

((3) November 20, 1981)

When Elsie asks for confirmation of her understanding of the situation, i.e., that the party will be at two in the morning, both the staff member and I replaced Elsie's lexical item *morning* with *afternoon* while accommodating to her syntactic structure. By using this strategy, we were able to get across the correct information without pointing directly through the use of *no* to Elsie's misunderstanding.

This type of response strategy, unlike the corrective and avoidance strategies just discussed, seems partially to carry out all three interactional goals at once. Coherence is established to a greater extent than in avoidance strategies, although arguably not to the degree of corrective strategies. Both Elsie's positive and negative face are protected, as I cooperate by giving her an answer (which is not the case with avoidance strategies) but simultaneously protect her negative face more than in corrective strategies by giving no direct signal of the problem. The approximate location of this strategy within the tridimensional space is accordingly represented by point C in figure 2.

Finally, if I do not wish to draw attention to the fact that I do not understand, but would like to make some linguistic contribution to the conversation, I can incorporate one or more of the lexical items in Elsie's utterance into my response. In this case, repetition of the other's words assists in faking understanding, which in turn helps to move the conversation along. In example 30, Elsie switches the topic with the question *Have they said anything what they're gonna do?* Although I have no idea who the referents for *they* are, I am able to transform Elsie's question into a negative response (*They haven't said anything*) followed immediately by what I wanted to say in the first place (*I'll just be here a few minutes*).

Example 30

ELSIE: Have they said anything what they're gonna do?
HEIDI: They haven't said anything but I'll just be here a few
    minutes.
ELSIE: Oh.
HEIDI: So we'll take you back.
ELSIE: All right. Sure. You'll just sit down for however long you
    want to.

((9) September 5, 1982)

It may be interesting to speculate here as to the reason I give a negative
rather than a positive response to Elsie's question when I actually have no
idea what she is talking about. It appears to relate to the grammatical fact
of English that only by responding in the negative could I use Elsie's word
anything. If I had responded in the affirmative, I would have had to say
Yes. They've said something and/or relay what was actually said. The
negative form of the response allows me to make an almost effortless link
to Elsie's question despite lack of understanding and to get on with my
own conversational goals. My incorporation of Elsie's words into my next
utterance simultaneously provides a cohesive response to her question as
well as a non-threatening one to her negative face by virtue of no explicit
reference to the communicative misunderstanding. These goals are fulfilled at the expense of overall coherence, as represented by point D in
figure 2.

Another example of this phenomenon comes from a conversation three
years later. In this situation Elsie has a runny nose and I am trying to offer
her a tissue (lines 1–3). In her next utterance (line 4), Elsie says *I know his
name*, probably in response to the last two words of my question, *your
nose* in lines 1–2 (note the phonological similarity between *your nose* and
you know his). Again, as in example 30, after making an effortless link to
Elsie's utterance in line 5, I get on with my own interactional goals (getting
Elsie to accept a tissue).

Example 31

1. HEIDI: Would you like a tissue for your
2.   nose? Would you like a Kleenex
3.   for your nose?
4. ELSIE: (Mhm). Oh yes. I know his name.
5. HEIDI: You know his name, but can I get you
6.   a Kleenex for your nose?

((12) July 4, 1985)

It is interesting to compare this strategy of repetition used by a "normal" interlocutor to give lip service to what the disabled individual said (without understanding it) and to get on with her own interactional goals with a strategy used by schizophrenics as described in Herbert and Waltensperger (1982: 237): "the situation in which a patient will respond to an interviewer's questions using many of the same words that the questioner has employed." Lehman (1980), as cited in Herbert and Waltensperger (1982: 238) suggests "that the patient, aware of his ideational shortcomings, uses this strategy as a compensatory mechanism in order to maintain a rapport with the interviewer."

As mentioned in chapter 1 of this study, Obler (1981: 379) has also noted the similarity between "normal" and "disabled" behavior in interviews. In her discussion of comments made by Irigaray (1973) which outline the language behavior of the examiner who is testing Alzheimer's patients, Obler notes that several of the experimenter behaviors Irigaray lists parallel the dementing behavior she describes elsewhere. These observations underscore once again the caution urged at the end of chapter 3 against setting up a strict dichotomy between "normal" and "disabled" individuals. We must find independent evidence which supports our different interpretations of the same phenomenon.

Example 32 illustrates the incorporation of both hybrid strategies (grammatical disagreement and other-repetition) just discussed in the design of a response when the misunderstanding appears to exist on the part of both interlocutors. In this interaction, I have just come to talk with Elsie for a little while. Because Elsie often seems unable to differentiate volunteers from residents of the center, I am confused when she combines the lexical item *stay* with *quite a while* in the design of her tag question, *You'll be staying here for quite a while then, won't you?* Does she think I have just moved into the center?

Example 32

> ELSIE: You've just drop . . just came?
> HEIDI: Yes I did. ⌐ Uhhuh . . uhhuh.
> ELSIE: └ Good. You'll be staying here for quite a while
>   then, won't you?
> HEIDI: Well, I come on Fridays and I stay for the exercise class
>   and then in the afternoon for the baking class.

((6) March 5, 1982)

My use of the verbs Elsie uses (*come, stay*) ties my utterance to her previous utterances, creating an illusion of understanding, while my use of the discourse marker *well* suggests that I am aware of my temporary inability to accomplish coherence (Schiffrin 1985). The fact that I change Elsie's use of tense (simple past for *come* and future continuous for *stay* in contrast to my use of the simple present for both verbs) allows me to emphasize that my actions are habitual; that is, that I come every week and stay for the classes every week, rather than having just arrived as a resident to live in the center for *quite a while*. The approximate location of this strategy within the tridimensional space is represented by point E, which takes into account the emphasis on positive and negative face and the somewhat offsetting consequences of the combined strategies with regard to coherence.

Which of the response strategies is chosen within the tridimensional space defined by relative focus on coherence, positive face maintenance, and negative face maintenance, then, seems to be influenced by the primary function of a given chunk of talk as perceived by the speaker. For example, if "reaffirming and strengthening relationships" (Lakoff 1973) is the primary purpose of the conversation, emphasis could be expected to be placed on face maintenance. Attention then would generally be directed towards positive or negative face depending on whether the "normal" speaker perceives independence or likability to be relatively more important to the conversational partner. On the other hand, if the "actual communication of important ideas" (Lakoff 1973) is the primary purpose, coherence would probably be emphasized to the detriment of face issues.

Elsie's inappropriate responses: caused by linguistic disability or motivated by face concerns?

Now that we have discussed the notions of coherence and positive and negative face maintenance as motivations underlying my choice of response strategy, it is time to turn to the question asked at the end of chapter 3, namely, are we justified in interpreting the same linguistic phenomenon in two different ways – one for the communicatively disabled individual and one for the "normal" individual? Are we not, in this case, judging a person to be communicatively disabled and then interpreting all of her verbal output from that perspective? And, if we do this, are we not excluding any possibility of finding that the disabled person does indeed use the same phenomenon as we do for the same purpose?

In this section, I make a first attempt to address this question. Before examining specific examples, it is important to provide some background on indirectness in conversation, i.e., how it is that listeners in general can understand what a speaker means when that meaning is different from the semantic meaning of the sentence uttered. For this kind of approach, we can turn to Grice's (1975) discussion of the Cooperative Principle assumed to be operative in conversations and its four maxims of quality ("be truthful"), quantity ("be sufficiently informative"), relation ("be relevant"), and manner ("be concise"). Briefly summarized, Grice argues that listeners are able to infer speaker meaning based on speaker deviations from these maxims. For example, when a speaker produces what the listener perceives to be an irrelevant utterance (or one which seems to be untruthful, provides insufficient information, or is overly wordy) and the listener assumes that the speaker is attempting to be cooperative in the interaction, then that listener infers (or, in Grice's terminology, draws an implicature) that the speaker means something other than what she actually said. An underlying assumption in this discussion of speaker meaning is that the speaker, by deviating from the maxims ("flouting" in Grice's terminology), *intended* her meaning to be different from the semantic meaning, and, additionally, *intended* her conversational partner to recognize this intention. This notion of intentionality will prove to be critical to the discussion of indirectness as it relates to language and Alzheimer's disease.

Now let us examine several of Elsie's inappropriate responses. In example 33 Elsie and I are looking at a silk-flower arrangement in her room. Elsie responds with a description of the flowers rather than answering my question as to whether or not she has had them a long time.

Example 33

HEIDI: Have you ⌐ had these a long time? ⌐
ELSIE: ⌐ yes ⌐ yes.
        Those are very pretty.

((9) September 5, 1982)

Example 34 takes place during my first visit to Elsie after my return from summer vacation.

Example 34

HEIDI: Do you remember me?
ELSIE: I've seen it I think I hope. But I don't know.

((9) September 5, 1982)

In this example, Elsie uses the [−human] personal pronoun *it* to refer to a person, me. The possibility that Elsie could be using *it* to refer to part of me (my face, for example) does not reduce the inappropriateness of her response. If she had wanted for some reason to refer to my face, she would have at least had to make a reference to me by saying, for example, *I've seen your face*. The grammatical mismatch between the [+human] pronoun *me* and the [−human] pronoun *it* underlies the inappropriateness of Elsie's response.

Example 35 comes from the same conversation as example 34. Since I had not talked with Elsie for a couple of months, I am trying to catch up on what Elsie has been doing since I last saw her.

> *Example 35*
>
> HEIDI: Did uh <u>have</u> you <u>been going</u> to exercise class? or to cooking class?
> ELSIE: <u>Tonight</u> you mean?
> HEIDI: With Jill, this summer. ⌜ Did you go?
> ELSIE: ⌞ Oh summer. Summer. There would be.

((9) September 5, 1982)

In this example, Elsie uses a temporal adverb referring to the *near future* (*tonight*) in response to my question in the *present perfect continuous* tense (*have you been going .. ?*).

Are the types of grammatical disagreement found in examples 33–35 different from the types of grammatical disagreement found in my responses? If so, how are they different? And is this difference justification enough to assign them different motivations? First of all, it is important to recognize that both Elsie's and my responses are syntactically well formed. In fact, most of these utterances would be completely appropriate in the right context, i.e., there is generally no syntactic or semantic disagreement *within* the utterances themselves. It is when one begins to examine Elsie's utterances *across turns* that the disagreement at various levels and the underlying linguistic disability become clear. It is only at the level of discourse that the complexity of the problem can begin to be sorted out.

Despite the fact that both Elsie and I appear to use the same response strategies in conversation and the fact that our utterances generally seem to be well-formed internally and would be judged to be grammatical sentences in isolation, there is one basic difference. This difference, I would argue, has to do with what can count in interaction as a *possible* motivation for using the more indirect, face-saving strategy instead of a direct strategy aimed at conversational coherence and, additionally, whether the speaker's intention connected with that motivation can be readily recognized by the listener. If the topic is very banal, such as Elsie's silk flowers as mentioned in example 33 above, it becomes very difficult for the ("normal") listener to imagine a possible situation which would warrant an indirect response. As cited in chapter 2, Brown and Levinson (1987: 268) suggest that this is a general problem of indirect uses of language: "Decoding the communicative intent relies on the mutual availability of a reasonable and particular motive for being indirect." I believe it is this difficulty in coming up with a possible motivation for using a face-motivated strategy which leads the listener to label a particular utterance as bizarre. If this utterance is not an isolated case, and if there is no indication from the speaker that the utterance is meant in jest, or that she is acting in an uncooperative fashion, this judgment of "bizarre" is transferred from the utterance to the speaker herself.

In chapter 2, it was suggested that Elsie's problem in understanding my indirectness as I had intended it to be understood is related to her problem in taking the role of the other, i.e., that she cannot understand my motivations for using indirectness when I do. I have just discussed my own inability to come up with possible motivations for Elsie's use of indirect-ness in certain cases (such as talking about her silk flowers). Although I used this problem on my part (as an interlocutor with no known language difficulties) as possible evidence that indirectness is not the motivating factor underlying Elsie's "inappropriate" responses, as it seems to be in my case, we cannot rule out the possibility Elsie is indeed motivated, as I am, by face concerns, but that she is "playing by different rules." The issue at the heart of this discussion is that of the researcher as relative insider/outsider. In any research project in which the researcher is not part of the population under examination, the danger exists that she will interpret an informant's behavior as if *she* herself were behaving that way. One linguistic form or communicative strategy may have a very different social meaning for one group than it has for another (see Gumperz 1982 for a discussion of this notion with regard to cross-cultural communication). As discussed in chapter 1, Smith and Ventis (1990) provide provocative evidence that Alzheimer's patients communicate differently with other Alzheimer's patients than they do with healthy friends, family members, and caregivers and, additionally, that they even give the impression of understanding other Alzheimer's patients better than these patients are understood by healthy interlocutors. Following the Gricean discussion above, the critical question here seems to be whether Elsie's "inappropriate" responses are actually cases of *intended indirectness* (and the motivations for that indirectness elude me as the listener, possibly because of my "outsider" status) or whether these responses are the result of the language breakdown associated with Alzheimer's disease and are therefore *unintended*.

In closing, even if it is the case that Elsie's inappropriate responses are primarily caused by language breakdown, this does not preclude the possibility that *some* of Elsie's choices of response strategies could be motivated by face concerns, nor does it preclude the possibility that *some* of my response types could be caused by other-than-face factors, such as tiredness or illness. Further detailed investigation would be necessary to determine the motivation in each individual case.

Summary

In this chapter we first set up the criteria for determining the appropriateness of a response to a question. These criteria, which were based on a close preliminary examination of Elsie's responses to my questions, allowed us to evaluate each response as being either fully appropriate or inappropriate in one of four ways. We then tracked Elsie's inappropriate responses over time and observed that (1) the changes which characterize Elsie's inappropriate responses over time are qualitative, rather than quantitative, ones, i.e., instead of the percentage of inappropriate responses increasing in each category over time, a different type of inappropriate response is prominent at different stages of the disease; and (2) in asking questions of Elsie over time, I accommodate to her increasing problems in responding, buoying up her performance in spite of these problems.

We then examined correlations between Elsie's appropriate and inappropriate responses and a variety of features of the questions which elicited these responses in an attempt to ascertain the relative influence of these question features on Elsie's ability to respond. We found, for example, that the grammatical type of question and its temporal reference seem to have more of an effect on Elsie's appropriateness of response than does the spatial reference of the question. Finally, focusing on the last taped conversation (March 1986) we saw evidence that Elsie's comprehension level may have been somewhat better than it had appeared at first blush due to her very limited production options.

In the second half of the chapter, I applied the appropriateness criteria developed for Elsie's responses to my own. Finding a small number of responses which would be classified as inappropriate according to these criteria, I delved deeper into the cause of this inappropriateness. These responses seemed to occur primarily in the face of a communicative breakdown. It seemed that in cases where I had not used a "before-the-fact" strategy, such as accommodation in my question design to prevent such a breakdown, I had to use an "after-the-fact" strategy in my response design ranging from avoidance to correction of the problem. This concern for face issues seemed to result in my use of "inappropriate" responses. I then discussed a tridimensional model within which such responses can be placed according to their relative focus on coherence and positive and negative face maintenance. A reexamination of Elsie's inappropriate responses was then necessary to determine whether her inappropriateness could also have been motivated by face concerns. There I found that lack of any possible face motivation (as determined by a "normal" interlocutor) generally justified the different interpretations of Elsie's and my "inappropriate" responses.

5   Conclusions and implications

In the fall of 1981, Elsie issued requests, expressed wishes, asked for information and clarification, expressed concern for others, provided excuses for her unexpected behavior, and refused offers – all by use of linguistic means. In the spring of 1986, she not once initiated an exchange verbally, but only responded to my utterances, agreeing with them (*mhm*), requesting repetition of them (*hmm?*), and expressing pleasure with them (*mmm*), all without using words. How did Elsie's abilities to use language to communicate change over these four-and-one-half years?

Here, just as in studies of historical linguistic change in the Labovian tradition (see Weinreich, Labov, and Herzog 1968; Labov 1972c), no individual stage in the breakdown of communicative abilities is static. We can expect to find evidence of dynamic language change at every point of our examination of language use. However, because of the relatively small number of many communicative phenomena in any given conversation in this data base, as well as the fact that these phenomena are not part of a closed set, it is not possible in most cases to determine exact percentages of use at each stage but only to note relative proportions of a feature or, in some instances, merely the presence or absence of a feature.

Changes in linguistic behavior can be either quantitative or qualitative; that is, in moving from one stage to another in a language loss situation, we can either find a steady increase (or decrease) over time in the occurrence of a particular phenomenon (quantitative change) or a shift in phenomena utilized in response to a particular communicative problem (qualitative change), such as responses to wh-questions or dealing with word-finding difficulties. By examining several of these individual stages over time, we can trace communicative breakdown both in qualitative and quantitative terms.

It is important here to point to a methodological problem inherent in studies of language loss, namely, how to determine the cause for the absence of a feature in a given conversation. Is Elsie actually unable to produce the feature in question or does she simply not produce it in *that* conversation? Although this is not so problematic in an examination of

148

those features for which *occurrence* marks a change from "normal" communicative competence (such as a yes–no answer to a wh-question), it is problematic for those for which *nonoccurrence* marks a change from the norm (such as self-initiated self-repair) – especially for those features which are less widespread in conversation in relation to others, such as account-giving as compared with turn-taking.

Despite this methodological difficulty, I still believe it is worthwhile to provide characterizations of Elsie's language use at various points in time over the four-and-one-half year period. In tracking the differences in the characterizations over time, we can observe which features appear to break down at the same time and which ones seem to be in a sequential relationship with each other. Following Obler's (1983: 271) recommendation: "It would be well worth studying the process of deterioration in order to discover the semiotic hierarchies of pragmatics," I offer the following characterization of four stages of Elsie's communicative abilities, recognizing that these are just snapshots and are only artificially distinct from each other. Following the prose characterization of each stage, I provide the reader with an extended excerpt from one of the conversations representing that stage. These transcriptions are intended to help the reader envision how the various communicative abilities and difficulties characterizing a given stage actually play out in a real-life interaction, although, of course, not all of the phenomena discussed in the prose characterization can be expected to be exhibited in any given conversational segment.

Stage 1: Active, confused, and aware

In this first stage of our interactions, Elsie is a very active participant both in terms of proportion of total number of words produced and in terms of proportion of total number of questions asked in each conversation. She is having trouble finding words in conversation, but frequently deals with this problem at this stage by providing a circumlocution or a semantically related word rather than a neologism, a word with a completely different lexical meaning, or an empty word, the three strategies she makes use of exclusively in later stages. Elsie is also having to deal with her problem in tracking the referents of pronouns used by others, although this is not obvious at the very beginning of this stage. She is generally aware of her memory problems at this time, as evidenced by her explicit reference to them. She seems to be aware of the unusualness of these problems with word-finding, reference, and memory, as she often provides excuses (although they are generally insufficient) for this unexpected behavior. She also recognizes when her abilities are unexpectedly good, as she provides explicit attests to these abilities and seems to be proud of them.

Elsie makes use of yes–no questions, including tag-questions, as well as of a full range of wh-questions to ask about the past, present, and future. She refers with her questions to persons, objects, and events both within and beyond her sight. Her inappropriate responses to questions are primarily grammatically mismatched and vague responses as compared with structural-level inappropriate responses or nonresponses. She uses a good deal of idiosyncratic ready-made language in the design of her conversational contributions, including the marked use of opposites, the marked use of the conditional mood (although not until later phases of this stage), and her own professional language from earlier in her life, as discussed in chapter 2. Despite some of the difficulties mentioned above, people generally enjoy talking with Elsie in this stage. Contributing to this overall ease in talk seems to be Elsie's use of positive politeness devices, such as compliments, expressions of appreciation to others, terms of endearment, and light-hearted jokes.

Example 1 begins approximately 5 minutes into a 31-minute conversation which took place on September 5, 1982. At this point in the conversation, Elsie and I were standing next to the chest of drawers in her room in the health care center.

> *Example 1* (September 5, 1982)
>
> 1. HEIDI: Do you want to explain some of these things to me?
> 2. [pointing to a variety of items, including figurines,
> 3. greeting cards, and framed photographs on top of her
> 4. chest of drawers]
> 5. ELSIE: Well yes. ⌐ [laughs —] This is .. This is .. Well this is
> 6. HEIDI: ⌐ [laughs] They look so pretty.
> 7. ELSIE: my husband ⌐
> 8. HEIDI: ⌐ That's your ⌐ husband ⌐
> 9. ELSIE: ⌐ (mine)   ⌐ Uhhuh. He's
> 10. (he's fine). ⌐
> 11. HEIDI: ⌐ He is. ⌐
> 12. ELSIE: ⌐ Yes. And we have a lot of papers
> 13. where they all where they have the different ones and look
> 14. up and take every uh carries on them of all kinds. And
> 15. these little [chuckles] kids. ⌐
> 16. HEIDI: ⌐ Yeah! ⌐ The little
> 17. ELSIE: ⌐ We've had those
> 18. arranged. Uhhuh. ⌐
> 19. HEIDI: ⌐ Uhhuh. ⌐ Those are cute. Who gave
> 20. ELSIE: ⌐ (Those are)

21. HEIDI: you those?
22. ELSIE: Well different ones. ⌐ Some of us. Some I did and
23. HEIDI: └ Uhhuh.
24. ELSIE: other people did.
25. HEIDI: I see.
26. ELSIE: And here's lots of em they've had on these to take em
27.   up. ⌐ And then we have the bit (sp pail) up here [points
28. HEIDI: └ Mhm.
29. ELSIE: up toward ceiling lamp]. I .. I'm not too uh
30. HEIDI: I think that's just a light.
31. ELSIE: Yes. ⌐ And
32. HEIDI: └ That's a light. ┐
33. ELSIE: └ Uhhuh. ┐
34. HEIDI: └ Uhhuh. ┐
35. ELSIE: └ And
36.   then uh. And uh. Yes. And it's espensive if you have to have
37.   use a whole lot of stuff, you know.
38. HEIDI: Right. A whole lot of light. Mhm.
39. ELSIE: So uh. But it works out nicely. And ⌐ these're
40. HEIDI: └ Sure.
41. ELSIE: These're these pretty little ones that go in ⌐ (there)
42. HEIDI: └ These
43.   are more flowers. ┐
44. ELSIE: └ Yes. Uhhuh. Aren't they darling?
45. HEIDI: Yes. ⌐ Well what is this? [pointing to photograph]
46. ELSIE: └ So we. So we fixed em up. We fixed em
47.   up. Well there I am. ⌐ And my my uh husband. ┐
48. HEIDI: └ Uhhuh. └ Oh
49.   how ⌐ cute.
50. ELSIE: └ And that uh is a good one.
51. HEIDI: That's a very good ⌐ picture. ┐
52. ELSIE: └ Uhhuh. └ Yeah. And we have.
53.   We had these up (wen) went out to the. Out when a when
54.   when they want to went out with the rest of em. ⌐ Where
55. HEIDI: └ Mhm
56. ELSIE: they had the batch of em on, you know. ┐
57. HEIDI: └ Mhm.
58. ELSIE: So and ⌐ there's stocking [pointing to a postcard].
59. HEIDI: └ Is that from a friend of yours?
60. ELSIE: That's stockings. Yes.
61. HEIDI: Mhm.

62. ELSIE: "Dear Elsie" and it says "I hope you" There's so
63. many here. Let's see. Uh "nee- needy" Uh that's
64. a little hard to write ⌐ those uh those ⌐
65. HEIDI: └ That's   └ Mhm. ⌐
66. ELSIE: └ thing.
67. Anyway. "I love you (nee nee) much. (Ell) I love.
68. Mary. ⌐ And uh name somebody else I forgot ⌐ who it
69. HEIDI: └ Mhm   └ Mhm
70. ELSIE: was ⌐ (with all the) you know when there's so many
71. HEIDI: └ Mhm
72. ELSIE: things ⌐
73. HEIDI: └ Oh right! ⌐
74. ELSIE: └ on you forget which one of
75.   ⌐ em it is [laughing] (to look. Mhm.)
76. HEIDI: └ Right.
77. HEIDI: This is your 40th anniversary picture.
78. ELSIE: Yes, I believe that's it. Uhhuh.

This segment shows Elsie to be an active participant in the conversation (1) by responding to my general question about a variety of items on top of her chest of drawers with comments about a family photograph (lines 5, 7, 9–10), greeting cards (lines 12–14), and porcelain figurines (lines 15, 17–18), (2) by responding to my question about a specific photograph (lines 45, 47–50), (3) by initiating conversation about the ceiling lamp in her room (lines 27–39) and some silk flowers in a vase (lines 41–44), and (4) by attempting to read a postcard which she had received from a friend (lines 62–75). Much of the difficulty in understanding Elsie's contributions is arguably due to the relatively unspecific nature of her utterances (e.g., "where they have the different ones," "you have to use a whole lot of stuff," "when there's so many things"). In this segment, her strategies in response to word-finding problems include not only relatively empty words, such as "stuff" for "electricity" or "light" in "It's espensive if you have to have use a whole lot of stuff, you know" (lines 36–37), but also semantically related terms, such as "write" for "read" in "That's a little hard to write" (lines 63–64), a word with a different lexical meaning, such as "stocking" presumably for "postcard" in "So and there's stocking" (lines 58). In this portion of the conversation, Elsie indicates not only that she is aware of her memory problems ("Somebody else I forgot who it was" – lines 68, 70) but also that such problems are unusual behavior which should be dealt with by providing an excuse for the behavior ("you know when there's so many things .. on you forget which one of em it is [laughing]" – lines 70, 72, 74, 75).

Stage 2: Active, confused, and unaware

In stage 2, Elsie continues to be an active participant in terms of proportion of total number of words produced in the conversations, but is much less active in producing questions in the interactions as compared with the first stage. It is more difficult to talk with Elsie now. This difficulty seems to stem in part from her decreasing awareness of her own communicative needs and those of others. In response to her word-finding problems, she no longer provides circumlocutions or semantically related words, but instead always provides either a neologism, an empty word, or a semantically unrelated word, options which are more difficult for the listener to "decode." Elsie no longer refers to her memory problems, nor does she provide excuses for her unexpected behavior. Her reference problems continue. She is beginning to repeat herself excessively (perseveration); when she does this, the repetition generally is of whole clauses rather than of individual words.

In terms of question production, Elsie continues to produce yes–no questions, including tag questions, and wh-questions (although no questions ask "who," "when," or "why"). The temporal reference of these questions continues to be to the past, present, and the future, although the spatial reference is now only to persons, objects, and events within her sight. Her inappropriate responses tend to be relatively evenly distributed among response types, although the proportion of responses deemed inappropriate because of being vague or grammatically mismatched is somewhat lower, and the proportion of structural-level inappropriateness is higher, than in stage 1. Elsie continues to use devices of positive politeness to make her conversational partner feel good, such as giving compliments, expressing appreciation, and telling jokes. She continues to make great use of the ready-made language she used in stage 1.

Example 2 begins approximately 10 minutes into a 38-minute conversation which took place on March 17, 1984 right before the evening meal. Throughout this conversation, Elsie and I were looking at and commenting on items in a mail-order catalogue which Elsie had with her.

Example 2 (March 17, 1984)

1. HEIDI: You must be almost ready to eat, huh?
2. ELSIE: Yes. ⌐ It is.
3. HEIDI: ⌐ You going to be eating? Mhm.

4. ELSIE: (I'll) say it is.
5. HEIDI: Uhhuh.
6. ELSIE: You can eat all you want.
7. HEIDI: You can eat all you want, huh?
8. ELSIE: Sure. ⌐ Yes (and I) ⌐
9. HEIDI: └ What ...   └ What do they have here to eat?
10. ELSIE: Yeah. And I put on some and keep and leave em, so
11.   they keep (right/write) it. And there will be on the
12.   (banquet) they come over, you know? There uh there's
13.   something here because we have more than other places
14.   (they have to close holes). So it's a crazy .. sometimes
15.   it's crazy. Now this is something here [turning
16.   attention back to the catalogue]. So now which is
17.   the most? Does that look like that is?
18. HEIDI: The most things to order? The most books here?
19. ELSIE: Oh yes. ⌐ Right here. Is that what you mean? Is
20. HEIDI: └ (They're) books.
21. ELSIE: that (take that out?)
22. HEIDI: These. Yeah. These are books that you can order.
23.   They're just showing them ... what they look like.
24. ELSIE: Mhm. Sure.
25. HEIDI: And then all the titles are here. ⌐ And the prices
26. ELSIE: └ Oh yes. That's
27. HEIDI: are here.
28. ELSIE: the (nissan). That's the (near sypay). And then.
29.   So is this. I have to take .. that there.
30. HEIDI: Mhm. There are books on a lot ⌐ of different ⌐ subjects.
31. ELSIE: └ There   └ there
32.   and there's (glen). There'll be one here. Right
33.   here. ⌐ And then there's another. ⌐ And so he'll have one.
34. HEIDI: └ Mhm.   └ Uhhuh.
35. ELSIE: And then that's gone ⌐ and the other man I don't
36. HEIDI: └ Mhm
37. ELSIE: know why. And this should be. Well we can probably
38.   send it ⌐ (and we've done this, see? for work working with
39. HEIDI: └ Mhm.
40. ELSIE: the darns)
41. HEIDI: Mhm.
42. ELSIE: So we can (kill) that. (Cause they don't think of that)
43.   And some of this some of this. ⌐ (And hard) taking care
44. HEIDI: └ Mhm.

45. ELSIE: of it. (Yeah. This is it. This'll be sure of it.)
46. HEIDI: Yeah. That's the end of the book.
47. ELSIE: Yeah. ⌈ That's right. Mhm.⌉
48. HEIDI: ⌊Mhm.   ⌊ Because it gives a list of
49. everything that's in there.
50. ELSIE: Now this is a (reswana). See, he's left that
51. much ⌉
52. HEIDI: ⌊ mhm
53. ELSIE: and now she wants to have more cause he's holding
54. it up ⌈ and it does look pretty good. (I don't matter) how
55. HEIDI:⌊ Uhhuh
56. ELSIE: much (how much in) ⌈ so you can stop on that and
57. HEIDI: ⌊ Mhm
58. ELSIE: choo: choose it and write write some of it (for you
59. orstal)
60. HEIDI: (You) can write it down . . on⌈that list.⌉
61. ELSIE: ⌊Yeah.   ⌊ Mhm. Sure.
62. HEIDI: I don't remember where it⌈ is, though.⌉
63. ELSIE: ⌊ Yeah   ⌊ (Terrible)
64. HEIDI: Where's the list? Oh here it is.⌈ Remember this
65. ELSIE: ⌊ Oh yes. That's
66. HEIDI: one?
67. ELSIE: right. Mhm. Well I think if this is about that we have
68. done. [Directs attention to a resident passing by]
69. Hello, dear.
70. RESIDENT: Hello.
71. ELSIE: How are you doing, dear? You come and (visit) if you
72. want to.

In example 2, Elsie is still actively participating, but, when compared with example 1, it is more difficult for the listener to understand her contributions to the conversation. Part of this difficulty can be traced to Elsie's frequent use of neologisms (e.g. "nissan" and "sypay" in line 28; "reswana" in line 50) and pronouns with no clear referents in the earlier portions of the conversation nor in the catalogue in front of us (e.g. "And so he'll have one" in line 33; "See, he's left that much and now she wants to have more" in lines 50–51, 53), as well as the lack of explicitly coherent ties between her responses and my questions (e.g. the structural mismatch of "what do they have here to eat?" and "Yeah. And I put on some and keep and leave em ..." in lines 9–10). An example of possible early perseveration can be found in lines 28–35 ("And then. So is this. I have to take . . . that there . . . And there's (glen). There'll be one here. Right here. And then there's another. And so he'll have one. And then that's gone."). Evidence of Elsie's continued use of positive politeness to reach out to other people can be found at the end of this segment (lines 66–69) as she greets a resident passing by ("Hello, dear. How are you doing, dear? You come and (visit) if you want to.")

Stage 3: Less active, confused, unaware

In stage 3, Elsie's participation in the conversations is markedly reduced, in terms of proportion both of total number of words and of question production, when compared with the first two stages. She continues to respond to her word-finding difficulties by using neologisms, empty words, and semantically unrelated words. She continues to have difficulty with reference. In terms of question production, Elsie no longer produces tag questions; the yes–no questions and wh-questions she uses (only *what?*, *how?*, and *which?*) refer only to the present time. The inappropriateness of her utterances in the response slot is now largely due to "non-response." She frequently repeats herself and others excessively (perseveration), often involving the repetition of a single lexical item, although at times she still uses self- and other-repetition appropriately. She continues to use questions appropriately to ask for clarification and occasionally repairs her own utterances. Ready-made language continues to be used in the design of her conversational contributions. Most of the evidence of positive politeness (with the exception of terms of endearment) which made talking with Elsie pleasant despite sense-making difficulties in the earlier stages is nowhere to be found in her discourse at this stage. Elsie no longer compliments or expresses interest in her conversational partner, nor does she express appreciation explicitly, or use humor or exclamatory questions. Elsie continues to use attention-getting techniques, request action from her conversational partner, state her own wishes, check her own understanding, make statements about some of her disabilities, express deference, and use metacommunicative framing utterances.

Example 3 begins approximately 10 minutes into a 29-minute conversation which took place on July 4, 1985. During this conversation, Elsie was in her room in bed and I was standing next to her.

Example 3 (July 4, 1985)

1. HEIDI: This is a pretty color on you. This looks pretty.
2. ELSIE: and what a (beautigo) ( ) have to go. and when
3. (yes . . yes) you you have a . . .
4. HEIDI: Are you trying to look at something?

5. ELSIE: No I wasn't uh finish.
6. HEIDI: You weren't finished.
7. ELSIE: I (can goes and mease class) . . Gee whiz (how) in it
8. cause. Let's see. You're you're str:. Let's see.
9. (They) they're they're (sudding) it.
10. HEIDI: Hmm?
11. ELSIE: (That's their s . .) here. I'm (host . .)
12. HEIDI: Are you looking outside?
13. ELSIE: (Na . . . .)
14. HEIDI: Hmm?
15. ELSIE: Yes.
16. HEIDI: Would you like a tissue for your nose? Would you
17. like a Kleenex for your nose?
18. ELSIE: (Mhm). Oh yes. I know his name.
19. HEIDI: You know his name, but can I get you a Kleenex for
20. your nose?
21. ELSIE: (Mace) and then and then now. And I don't know
22. what I . . I don't know what to (pick) [touching my purse]
23. HEIDI: Mhm. That's my purse.
24. ELSIE: Mhm.
25. HEIDI: Mhm.
26. ELSIE: (I don't know what. I don't know what to do.)
27. HEIDI: You don't want what?
28. ELSIE: I don't I don't think you'd better ( ) do that.
29. HEIDI: What don't you want? Hmm?
30. ELSIE: ( ) seeing ( )
31. HEIDI: Why don't I get you a Kleenex? I'll be right
32. back.
33. ELSIE: Yes ⌐ (and I'll think) . . I don't know why (that it's)
34. HEIDI: ⌐ Okay? [leaves to get Kleenex]
35. ELSIE: happening to (me).
36. HEIDI: [returns] Here's your Kleenex. Is that better?
37. ELSIE: Uh huh. Me me is is is on the (seat right here).
38. Gee it's it's uh (better get so sets) cause (there
39. another to go). Cause I want to know.
40. HEIDI: What do you want to know?
41. ELSIE: (Hmm?) Well that's (gallitzer cr crom). He is is
42. is is is his own ( ). See that here. Just as
43. (s:) help
44. HEIDI: The flower? This flower?
45. ELSIE: (knows how clo clothes)
46. HEIDI: What do you want? The clothes?

47. ELSIE: Yes.
48. HEIDI: Your clothes?
49. ELSIE: And I don't want to get ( ) and then (outside) and
50.   then (you were tea, you see)
51. HEIDI: I was what?
52. ELSIE: Yes. Uh (see you o o) in (trua) in five. And I I'm.
53. HEIDI: This is a. This is a nice magazine. (It's) a
54.   National Geographic magazine. Have you seen this?
55. ELSIE: I don't understand it .. stand it and (hand).
56. HEIDI: You don't understand the magazine? Would you like
57.   me to help you look at the magazine? See this is
58.   a man underwater with a big fish.

As example 3 shows, much of the difficulty in understanding Elsie's utterances has to do with her increased usage of neologisms (e.g. "They're they're (sudding) it" in line 9; "Well that's (gallitzer cr crom)" in line 41) and perseveration, both of clauses (e.g. "And I don't know what I .. I don't know what to (pick) . . . (I don't know what. I don't know what to do)" in lines 21–22, 26) and of individual lexical items (e.g. "Me me is is is on the (seat right here)" in line 37; "He is is is is is his own ( )" in lines 41–42). It is interesting to note, however, that Elsie still exhibits an awareness of her own decreased abilities (e.g., "I don't understand it .. stand it and (hand)" in line 55) and still asserts her wishes and opinions (e.g., "Cause I want to know" in line 39; "I don't I don't think you'd better ( ) do that" in line 28). Lines 7–9 provide clear evidence of Elsie's greater ability to use ready-made language (e.g., "Gee whiz" in line 7; "Let's see" in line 8) than the relatively incoherent utterances which surround the linguistic formulas (e.g., "I (can goes and mease class)" in line 7; "(how) in it cause" in lines 7–8.

Stage 4: Passive

In this stage, Elsie's participation level is even more markedly reduced than in stage 3. Now she produces no lexical items, her utterances being confined to the set of *uhhuh, mhm, mm Hm, mmm,* and *hmm?*. Elsie's responses to questions, then, are either appropriate if an affirmative answer or an action would be considered appropriate, or inappropriate because of non-response or question-type mismatch (affirmative answer to a wh-question). Despite her limited communicative repertoire, Elsie is still able to request repetition of her conversational partner's utterance (*hmm?*), to take conversational turns appropriately, and to indicate that she recognizes personally important topics (*mmm* and by specific actions).

Example 4 begins approximately 10 minutes into a 23-minute conversation which took place on March 18, 1986. During this conversation, Elsie was in her room in bed and I was standing at her side.

Example 4 (March 18, 1986)

1. HEIDI: Here I'll show you a picture. Hmm? Do you wanna
2. see a picture?
3. ELSIE: Mhm.
4. HEIDI: Yeah? I'll see if you know who this is. Just a
5. second. [leaves to get photograph and returns] Look
6. at this. Who's that?
7. ELSIE: Mmmmm. [high to low pitch contour]
8. HEIDI: Isn't that .. Is that a nice man?
9. ELSIE: Mhm.
10. HEIDI: Who is that?
11. ELSIE: Mhm.
12. HEIDI: Is that your husband? [leaves to get another
13. photograph and returns] Look at this one. Do
14. you know this person?
15. ELSIE: Mhm. Mhm.
16. HEIDI: [chuckles] That's you!
17. ELSIE: Mm Hm.
18. HEIDI: Right? Look at what a pretty dress you have on
19. in that picture!
20. ELSIE: Mhm [sniffles]
21. HEIDI: [leaves and returns] Oh-oh. ⌐
22. ELSIE: ⌐ Mhm. ⌐
23. HEIDI: ⌐ Yeah.
24. You've got a runny nose.
25. ELSIE: Mhm. Mhm.
26. HEIDI: Look at this! You used to always like to look at
27. these!
28. ELSIE: Mhm. Mhm. ⌐
29. HEIDI: ⌐ Uhhuh. ⌐
30. ELSIE: ⌐ Mhm. ⌐ [chuckles]
31. HEIDI: ⌐ National
32. Geographics.
33. ELSIE: Mhm.
34. HEIDI: Those are really good, huh?

35. ELSIE: Mm Hm.
36. HEIDI: Interesting pictures. Want to open it up and look at
37. it a little bit? Let's see what's in here. Oh boy.
38. Look at this big library. All these books. [Elsie and
39. Heidi look at that page; Heidi turns to new page]
40. Look at that. All sorts of fish. [Elsie and Heidi
41. look at new page]. Hmm. You're a sweet lady.
42. [chuckles]
43. ELSIE: Mmm ⌐ [chuckles].
44. HEIDI: ⌐ You are a sweet lady. ⌐
45. ELSIE: ⌐Mhm mmm.

In this segment, we see evidence of Elsie's ability to help maintain a conversation by her understanding of where to place her nonlexical utterances. This is perhaps especially evident in lines 26–40, where out of nine turns which deal with the topic of *National Geographic* magazines, 5 turns (4 by Elsie; one by me) consist solely of "mhm," "uhhuh," or "Mm Hm." Elsie's three tokens of "mmm" (which seem at this stage to be reserved for relatively emotional topics) in this segment are in response to seeing a photograph of her husband (lines 5–7) and to my telling her that she is a "sweet lady" (lines 41–45). Somewhat ironically, perhaps, because of her greatly reduced linguistic repertoire, Elsie's utterances at this late stage tend to be easier to understand, and a greater proportion of them are judged to be appropriate, when compared with the earlier three stages. (The one clearly inappropriate response in this segment can be found in lines 10–11: "Who is that?" "Mhm".) This is not to say that more substantive responses would not be expected from a healthy interlocutor; there is simply less that can go wrong in what Elsie produces at this late stage.

Of course, as we have seen throughout this study, the influence of one conversational partner on the language produced by the other conversational partner cannot be taken lightly. Portions of the characterizations of Elsie's communicative behavior at the four stages above, therefore, may be at least partially influenced by behavior on my part. These methodological concerns will be taken up in the sections that follow.

Implications

The present study has implications for (1) applications to diagnostic assessment and therapy, (2) the methodology of future studies of communicative breakdown and language loss, and (3) linguistic theory. These areas will be addressed in turn.

Application

Diagnostic assessment   One of the reasons I have chosen to focus on questions and responses in this study is because of their role in clinical assessments of Alzheimer's disease and other types of dementia. As I stated in chapter 3, what we learn about a patient's ability to ask and respond to questions in a relaxed, natural setting may help us to create more fitting and differentiated diagnostic tasks than exist at present. It is my hope that the findings of this study will prove to be useful to this end.

Following an investigation of additional Alzheimer's patients in a variety of interactional settings and any subsequent necessary revisions of the communicative breakdown sequence represented in the characterizations above, a set of questions and tasks could be devised to be used in the assessment regarding the level of the patient's current communicative ability and stage of the disease. Obviously here it would be most important to look for those features which Elsie stops using relatively early, as these will be more useful to us in differentiating stages than those features which are used throughout the conversations in my study. The following questions indicate how my findings could be operationalized.

(1) How does the patient handle a word-finding problem in natural conversation? Use of a circumlocution or semantically related word indicates an earlier stage; use of a neologism or unrelated word indicates a relatively later stage (although these do occur infrequently in early stages); use of an empty word is indeterminate.

(2) How does the patient handle a forgotten fact about his or her family or own life which should have been remembered? Use of a phrase such as *I forget* and/or an account of the "untoward" behavior indicates a relatively early stage. Absence of such an indication that the patient is aware of his or her memory problem may indicate a later stage.

(3) How does the patient react to his or her own exhibition of ability to remember something usually forgotten or to carry out a task usually not done? If the patient provides a metacommunicative attest to his or her ability, this indicates a relatively early stage.

(4) What kinds of questions does the patient produce within the natural setting? Wh-questions including the words "why," "who," "when," and "where" suggest an earlier stage, as does the formation of tag questions, and questions referring to persons, objects, and events not in sight. Because yes–no questions and wh-questions including the words "what," "how," and "which," which refer to the present time, continue to be used over a relatively long time, their occurrence cannot "flag" an early stage although, of course, they are used in early stages.

(5) How does the patient answer a wh-question? An inexplicit answer indicates an early stage; a full answer to a different wh-question than the one which was asked indicates a slightly later stage; a yes–no answer indicates a middle-to-late stage, and no response indicates a late stage.

(6) How does the patient interact with the interviewer or others in the ocnversation? Compliments, expressions of appreciation, requests for information about the conversational partner, or indications of a sense of humor are all characteristic of a relatively early stage. Lack of interest in the conversational partner accompanied by relatively high amount of interest in pursuing one's own needs and desires and fixed linguistic formulas may indicate a relatively late stage. The absence of any initiative behavior indicates a late stage in the disease.

(7) Is the patient's discourse characterized by an unusually high proportion of some specific feature which is not part of the culture's store of ready-made language? This use of (sometimes marked) individual ready-made language seems to characterize a relatively early stage, whereas use of more generally shared linguistic formulas characterizes later stages.

In his discussion of Mead, Cottrell (1980) points to the difficulty of operationalizing Meadian concepts for use in applications to problems of social life. The discussion in the present study of Mead's concept of "taking the role of the other" suggests a variety of levels on which the role of the other can be taken, such as in creating coherence, maintaining positive and negative face in interaction, and attending to structural concerns in conversation. This kind of approach can be helpful both to longitudinal studies in the future, such as in the examination of the "slow and progressive loss of self" in senile dementia suggested by Kitwood (1988: 176), and to studies contrasting dementia with other types of mental disability.

In the former case, it is likely that the identification of the gradual deterioration in degree and type of taking the role of the other could have consequences for assessment of the level of the disability. Emery (1988) has suggested that "the dementing process of Alzheimer's disease is also a process of desocialization because it strips the person of the capability of interacting according to socially prescribed patterns." The discussion of discourse-level manifestations of the decreasing ability to take the role of the other will help us to better understand the relationship between Alzheimer's patients' abilities to act as social beings and their performance of communicative abilities, more clearly outlining and operationally defining the social stages these patients pass through from the normal, socially interactive stage to a more ego-centered stage (see Hutchinson and Jensen 1980). The findings are also expected to illuminate the complex interdependence of decline as a social being and human cognitive decline. In the latter case, it is imaginable that various groups of mentally disabled individuals would have different degrees and types of abilities in taking the role of the other in conversation, which could have consequences for diagnosis. It is hoped that such longitudinal and contrastive studies will be able to elaborate upon the discussions in this study.

Therapy Given that the language problems characteristic of Alzheimer's disease are caused not by depression or the incorrect dosage of a particular medication (as some language problems are), but by irreversible (at least to date) physiological changes in the brain, is there any prospect of treating these language problems? Is any therapeutic approach available which can help Alzheimer's patients to deal better with their reduced linguistic abilities?

Barnes (1974) examined the effect of a six-week Reality Orientation[1] class on the level of confusion exhibited by six participants with senile dementia. Although pre- and post-period scores on a questionnaire indicated *no* significant improvement in the patients over the six-week time period, the nursing director responsible for the patients reported a number of important changes she and her staff had noticed in the patients at the end of the therapy program, such as greater interest in their environment, greater responsiveness and spontaneity, more hopeful attitudes, and greater cooperativeness. Barnes notes, however, that the behavioral improvement need not necessarily be linked to the class content *per se*, but might be attributable to the increased attention paid to the patients during the study. An earlier study of mine of the transition talk to and from a morning exercise class by twelve female nursing home residents indicated the same positive effect of the "therapy" session. Comparing topics introduced in assertions by the residents on the way to class with those introduced returning from class indicated that, following the class, the residents engaged in relatively more small talk, and talked more about their surroundings and less about themselves. When they did talk about themselves, they talked less about their wishes and needs and more about self-esteem. The activity's desired therapeutic effect appeared then to be reflected in the topics selected by the patients.

---

[1] Reality orientation therapy was developed beginning in 1959 to treat elderly patients with a moderate to severe degree of memory loss, confusion, and disorientation. This type of therapy aims to attack the deterioration process in two ways: (1) the patient is continually presented with basic information, such as the date, the location, and the weather; and (2) the therapy takes place in a group which gets the patient out of his or her isolated situation. (Information from Barnes 1974.)

Reisberg (1981: 149–150) recommends against the use of Reality Orientation, saying:

Attempting to educate and continually reeducate demented persons is probably of no value. However, befriending, communicating with, and comforting the senile is always appropriate ... A sensible, and truly humanitarian, approach to care would be to provide senile persons with the support which they require, depending upon their current capacities ... Just as for other human beings, a genuinely humanistic approach is one which aids in meeting a person's needs, desires, and aspirations and which respects the person's right to eschew that which, for whatever reasons, he or she would prefer not to face.

Wertz (1978) discusses a three-pronged approach to therapy for persons with Alzheimer's disease and related disorders which appears to be in harmony with the philosophy stated above: restitution of lost functions, reduction of the patient's need for functions that have been lost, and utilization of residual functions. "Although diseased neurons cannot be restored, efforts are employed to permit the neurons that are still functioning to perform optimally" (Wertz 1978: 59). Unfortunately, Wertz reports no significant improvement of an elderly male's communicative abilities (as measured by the Porch Index of Communicative Ability) following daily treatment over the period of one month.

Given the bleak outlook on actually improving the patient's communicative ability, it seems to me to be most reasonable to concentrate on Wertz's second and third points, i.e., to reduce the patient's need to use language abilities she no longer has and to utilize those which still exist. Before such an approach can be undertaken, however, these abilities and disabilities need to be identified. Once this has been done by means of a clinical assessment as described above, therapists and other persons close to the patient, such as nursing home staff and family members, will be able to take this information into account in the design of their talk to the patient. This more realistic set of expectations about the patient's communicative abilities will allow those who care for the patient to concentrate on tasks at the "appropriate" level, resulting in less frustration for all concerned. Of course, this does not preclude the possibility of exceptional moments when the patient can do more than she or he is expected to do. But these can be happy exceptions on the backdrop of reasonable expectations rather than long-awaited expected moments on the backdrop of frustration. Campbell-Taylor (1984) points out a potentially vital benefit of this approach to the patient: "Identifying ways in which they [Alzheimer's patients] appear to be less impaired and maximizing these can only improve the way in which they are regarded by others and, in turn, the way in which they are treated by them." In this way, both the patient and her conversational partner(s) can work together to construct a more positive social identity for the patient.

Methodological considerations

In the course of carrying out this study, at least three methodological considerations have arisen: (1) the necessity of creating a need to communicate as the basis for eliciting good discourse data; (2) the need to analyze the entire interaction, not just the patient's linguistic production; and (3) the problem of justifying same or different interpretations of similar behaviors by the "normal" interlocutor and the patient.

The case for natural data   Behind many observations regarding problems of Alzheimer's patients to communicate lie chunks of discourse which were elicited or strongly controlled by the researcher. For example, Obler (1981: 382) observes *no* occurrence in Irigaray's (1973) data of second-person pronouns, questions and commands, as well as lack of reference to the speaker as ego. When one looks at portions of transcript in other large studies, such as Bayles (1979, 1982) or Kempler (1984), these observations appear either to describe only the very latest stages of Alzheimer's disease or perhaps talk within a very limited setting.

The present study should serve to caution against using observations of conversations held in relatively artificial situations to draw conclusions about the patient's ability to communicate in everyday situations. When patients are not given the latitude to talk about topics of their own choosing or at their own pace, the resulting conclusions regarding their ability to use language creatively should be carefully considered. The descriptions may be of the barren, artificial interaction rather than of the patient's abilities.

Certainly there is a place for the type of testing of verbal expression and ability to repeat that is represented by example 5 from Bayles (1979). Here the subject is asked to talk about a common object, such as a button, and then to repeat what the researcher says. Much can be learned from such tests about topics such as phonological, syntactic, and semantic processing. But when we are trying to find out about the patient's ability to *communicate* with this linguistic knowledge, I would argue that we need to carry out the "test" in natural, symmetrical situations.

Example 5

E: Is it very big?
P: No, it's not very big. No, it's not very big.
E: What color is it?

P: Well, it's, it's not a black, and it's not exactly a brown, I don't
know what it is.

E: Say, "A little girl found a penny."

P: A little girl tore her heart.

E: Say, "The President lives in the White House."

P: The horse lives bright horse drawers.

(Bayles 1979: 128)

In the drill-like atmosphere of example 5 it would seem to be difficult for
the patient to undertake any communicative initiative or attempt to attain
any communicative goal. In order to attain this vital information on
interactive abilities, a different kind of research procedure is necessary. We
cannot expect patients to show us their full repertoire of communicative
abilities in the absence of a real need to communicate. It is only by
creating an environment in which a need to communicate can naturally
evolve that we can aim at seeing "a being conducting itself spontaneously
in its own natural way" (Sacks 1987: 181). In the design of future studies
of Alzheimer's patients' communicative competence, then, we must aim at
symmetry in the interaction. It is only when we depart from an interview
situation which is strictly controlled by the researcher that we will allow
the patient to show more of his or her communicative repertoire, his or her
abilities as well as deficits.

A conversational segment as part of a test battery may be more or less
successful in eliciting natural language from the patient depending on how
it is integrated into the rest of the battery. It may, for example, be signaled
solely by the examiner ("Okay, now let's just talk a bit, shall we?") or it
may take place at a more natural break in the test battery. The switching
of frames from a relatively free-flowing conversational segment to tests of
specific linguistic and cognitive abilities may make it difficult for the
patient to assess when her answer is really *needed* to fill a gap in the
clinician's knowledge and when it is only serving to point to abilities or
lack thereof on the part of the patient (as in the use of test questions to
which the examiner already knows the answer and is trying to determine
whether the patient does as well). We know from previous studies (Obler
1981; Appell, Kertesz, and Fisman 1982) that many Alzheimer's patients
are "context-bound." They may, therefore, have difficulty identifying and
following the breaks in frame if an examiner is in control of these breaks
from "test situation" to "natural conversation" and then from "natural
conversation" back to "test situation." From this perspective, perhaps a
patient's nonresponse to a test question is not caused only by linguistic
deficit, but by not understanding why the question was asked. As Crystal
(1984: 108) says, "seeing a reason for a question is often part of the

information needed in order to know how to answer." Given this situation, then, it is likely that incorporating a conversational component at a more natural break in the testing would be relatively more successful in eliciting natural language from an Alzheimer's patient than a break in frame signaled solely by an examiner's utterance. This approach has been used by Ripich, Vertes, Whitehouse, Fulton, and Ekelman (1991), who collected conversational language data during a coffee/tea break in the overall test situation.

Accommodation of the "normal" interlocutor to the patient As we saw in chapters 3 and 4, the role of the "normal" conversational partner cannot be ignored in analyses of patient discourse. Chapter 3 showed that Elsie produced fewer questions which refer to the present time than I did, as well as fewer what-questions which refer to concrete objects than to abstract objects and actions, and fewer tokens of the formulaic expression *how are you?* than other how-questions. It appeared that I was designing questions to match my *perceptions* of Elsie's linguistic and cognitive abilities which do not match her production abilities. Chapter 4 showed how I accommodated to Elsie's decreasing ability to answer questions over time by asking increasingly large numbers of yes–no questions and correspondingly low numbers of wh-questions during the last conversations. This unintentional adjustment strategy allowed Elsie, *despite decreasing abilities*, to continue to give a high proportion of appropriate answers to my questions.

These kinds of observations recommend strongly against a one-sided analysis of the interaction which examines the patient's language only. As we have seen in this study, the conversational partner's accommodations to the patient's language ability (or as it is perceived by the partner) can steer the interaction in a direction which suggests better or worse abilities on the part of the patient than actually exist. In the first case, adjustment on the part of the normal interlocutor in question strategy (such as question type and function) can result in better than expected answers by the patient. In the latter case, concentration on the "here and now" by the normal interlocutor may conceal the patient's abilities to talk about other times and places, lending the entire interaction an unnecessary air of context-boundedness. It is imperative that the conversational partner's language be examined as well as the patient's, so as to be able to assess its influence on the patient's performance.

Additional evidence of this phenomenon comes from Ripich, Vertes, Whitehouse, Fulton, and Ekelman (1991), which reports on an examiner's talk with Alzheimer's patients and compares it with that used by the examiner with normal elderly individuals. With regard to turns-at-talk, Ripich *et al* found that the examiner used fewer words per turn with the patients than with the normal elderly controls. They suggest that these briefer turns may be in response to the memory problems of the patients and allow for better "management of the conversation by the examiner" (Ripich *et al.* 1991: 340). Perhaps more important to the point here is their finding that the examiner asked more "process questions" (which seek extended descriptions or explanations) of the normal elderly controls than of the Alzheimer's patients, and, conversely, that she issued more action requests of the patients than of the normal elderly. This differential behavior toward the two groups of subjects may "reflect differing discourse expectations ... on the part of the examiner" (Ripich *et al.* 1991: 340).

   Need to justify varied interpretations of the same phenomenon   In the process of analyzing my responses to Elsie's questions just as I had analyzed Elsie's responses to my questions to determine their appropriateness, I determined that a number of my responses were inappropriate according to the criteria used to judge Elsie's responses. While I had been assuming that decreasing communicative abilities related to Alzheimer's disease were the reason behind Elsie's inappropriate responses, I could not very well use that reason to explain my inappropriateness. Further examination suggested that my "inappropriate" responses were motivated by my desire to save mutual face in the interaction. I stood before a problem. How could I say that my "inappropriate" responses were motivated by face concerns and insist without further examination that Elsie's "inappropriate" responses were actually inappropriate due to communicative breakdown? My subsequent analyses to determine whether Elsie may indeed have been motivated by face concerns in designing her inappropriate responses uncovered a difference in our responses. The perceived lack of possible motivation for face concerns in Elsie's responses made it unlikely in most cases that Elsie was acting out of concern for mutual face, although, as was mentioned in chapter 4, we cannot rule out that possibility that, as an outsider, I was unable to recognize her motivations.

   The point here is not whether different interpretations of the same (or similar) linguistic phenomenon turn out to be justified. Rather, my point is that we are running the risk of reporting self-fulfilling prophecies if we do not carefully check the possibility that the patient is operating under the same rules as we are. Otherwise, we may fall into the trap of interpreting every "suspicious-looking" phenomenon we encounter as a pathological feature to be used as further evidence to support what we already know. To aim at a balanced account, we should look for similarities as well as differences in communicative abilities of all concerned in the interaction and be ready to report the patient's strengths as well as her weaknesses.

Linguistic theory

In addition to clinical and methodological considerations, it is my hope that observations in this study will prove helpful to future considerations within discourse analysis and regarding the view of language in general. In their work on cross-cultural communicative breakdowns, Gumperz and Tannen (1979) point out that much knowledge can be gained regarding how "normal," everyday discourse works by trying to understand instances where it does not work so well. In his useful discussion of the ways in which analysts can "learn to notice what we normally take for granted" in social interactions, Stubbs (1983: 238) notes the effectiveness of concentrating on the causes, forms, and effects of miscommunication as a way of gaining insight into the routine structures of behavior. Both Obler (1981: 385–386) and Ulatowska, Allard, and Chapman (1990: 181) suggest the appropriateness of examining the dissociation between intact and impaired mechanisms underlying discourse produced by Alzheimer's patients as one way to gain insights into normal discourse processing.

This dissociation between intact and impaired mechanisms must exist, however, in this kind of examination. Menn and Obler (1982) argue that cases of complete breakdown are as little instructive as cases of normal performance are. The crucial cases for gaining information about a linguistic structure or discourse mechanism are those in which some partial performance is evidenced by an error of substitution which appears to have been constrained by that structure or mechanism. Examples of this kind of partial performance as evidenced in the present study include the variety of inappropriate responses which indicate different types of knowledge an interlocutor has about question/response pairs – beginning at the most basic level with the fact that one needs to respond in some way to a question, more specifically matching question and response type, then matching grammatical categories, and, finally, giving information specific enough to serve satisfactorily as an answer to the question.

Along this line, the more detailed understanding of the hierarchical relationships among a variety of linguistic phenomena as determined by the order of their breakdown in communication may be able to shed new light on pragmatic patterning in normal interlocutors as well as point to possible pragmatic universals gleaned from comparisons with other language loss and first language acquisition findings.

Additionally, it is hoped that future studies will be assisted by the contextualized discussions of taking the role of the other in conversation, division of labor in discourse, automaticity of language, as well as the tri-dimensional interactional model of response strategies, in terms of the role these play in maintaining successful interaction. The frameworks of taking the role of the other, as discussed in chapter 2, and division of labor in discourse, as discussed in chapter 3, allow us to work the critical element of intersubjectivity into our analyses of communicative break-down. The tridimensional space defined by relative amount of focus in response strategies on the interactional goals of coherence, positive face maintenance, and negative face maintenance, as discussed in chapter 4, goes beyond this consideration of intersubjectivity within situations of communicative breakdown. It allows us to further specify the shape that intersubjectivity takes in the design of a response to such a breakdown, taking into account how interlocutors resolve their desires to get across their message on the propositional level without sending the wrong message to either their partner's positive or negative faces.

Turning to the view of language in general, the observations made in this study regarding Elsie's language lend support to the vision of Becker (1984), Bolinger (1961, 1976), Hopper (1988) and Tannen (1987a) of language as relatively prepatterned rather than novel. From this perspec-tive, speakers do not actively create much (or most) of what they say, but rather "reach for" (Bolinger 1961: 381) prefabricated pieces which exist in an ever-growing inventory of talk they have used or heard before. This view not only accounts for the relatively high occurrence of recurring chunks of discourse in Elsie's speech; in emphasizing the individual's prior experience and access to prior texts, it also accounts for Elsie's continuing use of language from her earlier professional years, which is strikingly more intact than the language surrounding it. In addition, this view is supported by patient responses in confrontation-naming tasks which seem to relate personal experiences sparked by the experimental object rather than the linguistic label for it. As was reviewed in chapter 1, Bayles (1979) reports several instances of this phenomenon, one such example being the question *Where is the baby?* rather than the lexical item *matches* in response to a picture of matches.

The access to these accumulated prior texts, which Becker maintains *is* our real linguistic competence (Becker 1984: 435), is provided by our memory. In her discussion of "grammar as memory," Tannen (1987a: 218) maintains that linguists with this view of language "assign a much larger role to memory in the production of language: memory for the innumerable instances of language that have previously been heard." Along this line, Gleason (1982: 355) suggests that "linguistic models need to make room for memory." But what happens when memory begins to fail and an individual's access to earlier texts is slowly but surely cut off? What types of language hold on for relatively shorter or longer periods of time as memory fades? The observations made in chapter 2 and repre-sented in the characterization of the stages of Elsie's communicative abilities above can provide us with some answers to these questions. Generally, those linguistic abilities which are relatively more automatic remain intact longer than those more effortful, creative abilities. For example, Elsie uses culturally shared linguistic formulas long after she stops designing linguistic accounts for her inappropriate behavior.

Citing the important role which formulaic aspects of language play in a wide variety of domains, including rituals of law and religion, traditional oral literature, language acquisition, and language used by aphasic and dementing patients, Menn and Obler (1982: 8) state that "linguistic theory must deal with language as a continuum from the most creative to the most stereotypic communication." Tannen (1987a, 1987b) differentiates the notion of prepatterning in language even further. Of the three dimensions she discusses within which an utterance can be seen as prepatterned (form, context, and time), the continuum of relative fixity versus ephemerality over time seems to be most relevant to an explanation of the breakdown sequence in the present study, as was illustrated in chapter 2. At one end of this continuum are highly fixed, culturally shared sayings which are long-lived. At the other end are instances of repetition which are short-lived. Both types of prepatterned language, Tannen argues, are automatic and less energy-draining than novel language production. In looking at Elsie's conversational contributions, it seems to be the case that culturally shared formulas are relatively immune to memory problems, as is her ability to repeat an utterance made by her conversational partner (she does seem, on the other hand, to have problems with responding with an appropriate self-repetition to requests for such a repetition made by her interlocutor (*Hmm?*)). In between these two poles of long- and short-lived prepatterned language, memory problems seem to take their toll. As we saw above, it appears that Elsie stops using the prepatterned language which had derived more from her individual experiences before prepatterned language which is more short-lived, such as repetition in conversation, or long-lived, such as culturally shared formulaic expression.

Tannen argues that automaticity need not mean a move away from individual freedom, but that it is indeed necessary to achieve that freedom. Even in a case such as Elsie's, where the data show the clear tension between automaticity and autonomy as discussed in Sacks (1987: 39), automatic language frees her up in at least the following ways: (1) automatic language comprises a large amount of what Elsie can say clearly enough so that the conversational partner can understand it and will be encouraged to continue the conversation; (2) culturally important formulas (e.g., *How are you?*) provide relatively effortless outward evidence that Elsie is still a social being worthy of being involved in conversation; (3) Elsie's ability to repeat what her partner just said (short-lived prepatterned language) provides Elsie with additional vocabulary in the face of word-finding difficulties; and (4) to the extent that it contains words which she has automatized, Elsie seems more capable of correctly reading written passages aloud.

As was stated in the introduction to this book, Alzheimer's disease is a degenerative brain disease which has major social consequences for the individual who has the disease as well as for those who are emotionally and/or physically close to this individual. In the present study we have looked in some detail at the language used by one patient in natural conversations over four-and-one-half years. The preceding pages are full of evidence that the progression of Alzheimer's disease is accompanied by increasing difficulties in communicating. No one would deny this fact. What I have attempted to show here, however, is how something as highly personal as degenerative brain disease has interpersonal ramifications, in other words, to illustrate Crystal's (1984: 55) point that language handicap is "first and foremost an interactive phenomenon." This interactional sociolinguistic approach to one particular case of Alzheimer's disease should serve as one step toward understanding some of the ways in which an individual's language pathology can play itself out in interactions, how indeed the affected individual's relative successes in communicating are influenced by both preemptive and reactive communicative behaviors of the patient's healthy interlocutors.

This "personal and particular" (Becker 1988) study of conversations with one Alzheimer's patient is offered as a humanistic approach to language loss, one in which communicative breakdowns are analyzed not apart from details about the patient, her conversational partners, and the setting, nor from relevant social facts which may influence the interactions – one in which language is seen as an integral part of human life.

References

Agency for Health Care Policy and Research. 1987. *National Medical Expenditures Survey*. US Department of Health and Human Services.

Ajuriaguerra, J. de and Tissot, R. 1975. Some aspects of language in various forms of senile dementia (comparisons with language in childhood). In E. H. Lenneberg and E. Lenneberg (eds.), *Foundations of Language Development: a Multidisciplinary Approach*, 323–339. New York: Academic Press.

Alzheimer, A. 1907. Über eine eigenartige Erkrankung der Hirnrinde. *Allgemeine Zeitschrift für Psychiatrie* 64: 146–148.

Andresen, H. 1985. Selektiv erhaltene sprachliche Fähigkeiten bei schwerer Aphasie. In H. Andresen and A. Redder (eds.), *Aphasie: Kommunikation von Aphatikern in Therapiesituationen*, 43–69. Osnabrück: OBST32.

1986. Sagen können, dass man nichts sagen kann: Untersuchungen zur Funktion der Stereotypien in der Sprache eines schwer gestörten Aphasikers. In R. Mellies, F. Ostermann, and F. Vauth (eds.), *Erschwerte Kommunikation und ihre Analyse*. Hamburg: Helmut Buske Verlag.

Appell, J., Kertesz, A., and Fisman, M. 1982. A study of language functioning in Alzheimer patients. *Brain and Language* 17: 73–91.

Austin, J. L. 1962. *How to Do Things with Words*. Cambridge, MA: Harvard University Press.

Baltes, M. M. 1991. Dependency and successful aging: two sides of behavioral dependency. Paper presented at the 44th Annual Scientific Meeting of the Gerontological Society of America, November 22–26. San Francisco.

Barnes, J. 1974. Effects of reality orientation classroom on memory loss, confusion, and disorientation in geriatric patients. *The Gerontologist*, April 1974, 138–142.

Bayles, K. A. 1979. Communication profiles in a geriatric population. Unpublished Ph.D. dissertation. Tucson, Arizona: University of Arizona.

1982. Language function in senile dementia. *Brain and Language* 16: 265–280.

1984. Language and dementia. In A. Holland (ed.), *Language disorders in Adults: Recent Advances*, 209–244. San Diego, CA: College-Hill Press.

1985. Communication in dementia. In H. Ulatowska (ed.), *The Aging Brain*, 157–173. San Diego, CA: College-Hill Press.

Bayles, K. A., C. K. Tomoeda, A. W. Kaszniak, L. Z. Stern, and K. K. Eagans. 1985. Verbal perseveration of dementia patients. *Brain and Language* 25: 102–116.

Bayles, K. A. and Kaszniak, A. 1987. *Communication and Cognition in Normal Aging and Dementia*. Boston: Little, Brown and Company.

Becker, P. 1984. The linguistics of particularity: interpreting superordination in a Javanese text. *Proceedings of the Tenth Annual Meeting of the Berkeley Linguistics Society*, 425–436. Berkeley, CA: University of California.

1988. Language in particular: a lecture. In D. Tannen (ed.), *Linguistics in Context*. Norwood: Ablex.

Blakar, R. M. 1985. Towards a theory of communication in terms of preconditions. In H. Giles and R. N. St. Clair (eds.), *Recent Advances in Language, Communication, and Social Psychology*, 10–40. London: Erlbaum.

Blanken, G., Dittmann, J., Haas, J.-C., and Wallesch, C. W. 1987. Spontaneous speech in senile dementia and aphasia: implications for a neurolinguistic model of language production. *Cognition* 27: 247–274.

Bolinger, D. 1961. Syntactic blends and other matters. *Language* 37: 366–381.

1976. Meaning and memory. *Forum Linguisticum* 1: 1–14.

Boller, F., Cole, M., Vrtunski, P. B., Patterson, M., and Kim, Y. 1979. Paralinguistic aspects of auditory comprehension in aphasia. *Brain and Language* 7: 164–174.

Bowen, D. M. 1987. Cell injury: molecular biology and genetic basis. Group report 3 of the Dahlem Workshop on the Etiology of Dementia of Alzheimer Type. December 7–11. Berlin.

Brown, P. and Levinson, S. 1978. Universals in language usage: politeness phenomena. In E. Goody (ed.), *Questions and Politeness*, 56–289. Cambridge University Press.

1987. *Politeness: Some Universals in Language Usage*. Cambridge University Press.

Brown, G. and Yule, G. 1983. *Discourse Analysis*. Cambridge University Press.

Campbell-Taylor, I. 1984. Dimensions of Clinical Judgment in the Diagnosis of Alzheimer's Disease. Unpublished Ph.D. dissertation. Buffalo, NY: State University of New York.

Caporeal, L. 1981. The paralanguage of caregiving: baby talk to the institutionalized aged. *Journal of Personality and Social Psychology* 40: 876–884.

Caramazza, A. 1986. On drawing inferences about the structure of normal cognitive systems from the analysis of impaired performance: the case for single-patient studies. *Brain and Cognition* 5: 41–66.

1991. Data, statistics, and theory: a comment on Bates, McDonald, MacWhinney, and Applebaum's "A maximum likelihood procedure for the analysis of group and individual data in aphasia research." *Brain and Language* 41: 43–51.

Caramazza, A. and Badecker. 1989. Patient classification in neuropsychological research. *Brain and Cognition* 10: 256–295.

Causino, M., Obler, L., Knoefel, J., and Albert, M. (forthcoming). Pragmatics in end-stage dementia of Alzheimer's disease. In R. Bloom, L. Obler, S. De Santi, and J. Ehrlich (eds.), *Discourse in Adult Clinical Populations*.

Clark, E. O. 1980. Semantic and episodic memory impairment in normal and cognitively impaired elderly adults. In L. Obler and M. Albert (eds.), *Language and Communication in the Elderly*, 47–57. Lexington, MA: Lexington Books.

Cottrell, L. S. 1980. George Herbert Mead: The legacy of social behaviorism. In R. K. Merton and M. White Riley (eds.), *Sociological Traditions from Generation to Generation*, 45–65. Norwood, NJ: Ablex.

Coulthard, M. 1977. *An Introduction to Discourse Analysis*. London: Longman.

Coupland, N., Coupland, J., Giles, H., and Henwood, K. 1988. Accommodating the elderly: invoking and extending a theory. *Language in Society* 17: 1–41.

Coupland, N., Coupland, J., and Giles, H. 1991. *Language, Society and the Elderly*. Oxford: Blackwell.

Coupland, J., Coupland, N., and Grainger, K. 1991. Intergenerational discourse: contextual versions of ageing and elderliness. *Ageing and Society* 11: 189–208.

Coupland, N., Giles, H., and Wiemann, J. (eds.). 1991. *"Miscommunication" and Problematic Talk*. Newbury Park: Sage Publications.

Crystal, D. 1984. *Linguistic Encounters with Language Handicap*. Oxford: Blackwell.

Cummings, J., Houlihan, J., and Hill, M. 1986. The pattern of reading deterioration in dementia of the Alzheimer type: observations and implications. *Brain and Language* 29: 315–323.

Cuzzort, R. and King, E. 1980. *20th Century Social Thought*, 3rd edition. New York: Holt, Rinehart, and Winston.

De Santi, S., Obler, L., Sabo-Abramson, H., and Goldberger, J. 1990. Discourse abilities and deficits in multilingual dementia. In Y. Joanette and H. Brownell (eds.)., *Discourse Ability and Brain Damage*, 224–235. New York: Springer Verlag.

Edgerton, R. 1967. *The Cloak of Competence: Stigma in the Lives of the Mentally Retarded*. Berkeley: University of California Press.

Emery, O. 1988. Language and memory processing in senile dementia Alzheimer's type. In L. Light and D. Burke (eds.), *Language, Memory, and Aging*. Cambridge University Press.

Erickson, F. 1986. Listening and speaking. In D. Tannen (ed.), *Languages and Linguistics: The Interdependence of Theory, Data, and Application GURT 1985*, 294–319. Washington, DC: Georgetown University Press.

Evans, D. *et al.* 1990. Estimated prevalence of Alzheimer's disease in the United States. *The Milbank Quarterly* 68: 267–289.

Figurski, T. 1987. Self-awareness and other-awareness: the use of perspective in everyday life. In K. Yardley and R. Honess (eds.), *Self and Identity: Psychosocial Perspectives*, 197–210. Chichester: John Wiley & Sons.

Flicker, C., Ferris, S., Crook, T., and Bartus, R. 1987. Implications of memory and language dysfunction in the naming deficit of senile dementia. *Brain and Language* 31: 187–200.

Fromm, D. 1988. Language and Memory in Alzheimer's Disease: A Study of Functional Skills. Unpublished Ph.D. dissertation. University of Pittsburgh.

Fromm, D. and Holland, A. 1989. Functional communication in Alzheimer's disease. *Journal of Speech and Hearing Disorders* 54: 535–40.

Gardner, H. 1974. *The Shattered Mind: The Person After Brain Damage*. New York: Random House.

Garfinkel, H. 1972. Remarks on ethnomethodology. In J. Gumperz and D. Hymes (eds.), *Directions in Sociolinguistics*, 301–324. New York: Holt, Rinehart and Winston.

176 *References*

Garvey, C. 1977. The contingent query: a dependent act in conversation. In M. Lewis and L. Rosenblum (eds.), *The Origins of Behaviour*. New York: Wiley.
  1979. Contingent queries and their relations in discourse. In E. Ochs and B. Schieffelin (eds.), *Developmental Pragmatics*. New York: Academic Press.
Gleason, J. B. 1982. Converging evidence for linguistic theory from the study of aphasia and child language. In L. Obler and L. Menn (eds.), *Exceptional Language and Linguistics*, 347–356. New York: Academic Press.
Goffman, E. 1961. On the characteristics of total institutions. In Goffman, *Asylums*, 1–124. Garden City, NY: Doubleday.
  1963. *Stigma: Notes on the Management of Spoiled Identity*. Englewood Cliffs, NJ: Prentice-Hall, Inc.
  1967. On face-work. In Goffman, *Interaction Ritual*, 5–45. Garden City: Doubleday.
  1981. Replies and responses. In Goffman, *Forms of Talk*, 5–77. Philadelphia: University of Pennsylvania Press.
Golper, L. and Binder, L. 1981. Communication behavior in aging and dementia. In J. Darby (ed.), *Speech Evaluation in Medicine*, 166–167. New York: Grune and Stratton, Inc.
Goodglass, H. and Kaplan, E. 1972. *Assessment of Aphasia and Related Disorders*. Philadelphia: Lea and Febiger.
Goody, E. (ed.). 1978. Towards a theory of questions. *Questions and Politeness*, 17–43. Cambridge University Press.
Grafman, J., Thompson, K., Weingartner, H., Martinez, R., Lawlor, B., and Sunderland, T. 1991. Script generation as an indicator of knowledge representation in patients with Alzheimer's disease. *Brain and Language* 40: 344–358.
Grice, H. P. 1975. Logic and conversation. In P. Cole and J. L. Morgan, *Speech Acts*, Syntax and Semantics, vol. III, 41–58. New York: Academic Press.
Gumperz, J. (ed.). 1982. *Language and Social Identity*. Cambridge University Press.
Gumperz, J. and Tannen, D. 1979. Individual and social differences in language use. In C. Fillmore, D. Kempler and W. S.-Y. Wang (eds.), *Individual Differences in Language Ability and Language Behavior*, 305–325. New York: Academic Press.
Halliday, M. A. K. 1978. *Language as Social Semiotic*. London: Edward Arnold.
Halliday, M. A. K. and Hasan, R. 1976. *Cohesion in English*. London: Longman.
Hamilton, H. 1988. Causes and consequences of communicative breakdown: The case of Alzheimer's disease. *Linguistische Berichte* 113.
  1991. Accommodation and mental disability. In H. Giles, J. Coupland, and N. Coupland (eds.), *Contexts of Accommodation: Developments in Applied Sociolinguistics*, 157–186. Cambridge University Press.
  forthcoming. Requests of clarification as evidence of pragmatic comprehension difficulty. In R. Bloom, L. Obler, S. De Santi, and J. Ehrlich (eds.), *Discourse in Adult Clinical Populations*.
Henderson, V., Mack, W., Freed, D., Kempler, D., and Anderson, E. 1990. Naming consistency in Alzheimer's disease. *Brain and Language* 39: 530–538.
Herbert, R. K. and Waltensperger, K. Z. 1982. Linguistics, psychiatry, and psychopathology: the case of schizophrenic language. In L. Obler and L.

Menn (eds.), *Exceptional Language and Linguistics*, 217–246. New York: Academic Press.

Hier, D., Hagenlocker, K., and Shindler, A. 1985. Language disintegration in dementia: effects of etiology and severity. *Brain and Language* 25: 117–133.

Hopper, P. 1988. Emergent grammar and the *a priori* grammar postulate. In D. Tannen (ed.), *Linguistics in Context*. Norwood: Ablex.

Huff, F. Jacob, Corkin, S. and Growdon, J. H. 1986. Semantic impairment and anomia in Alzheimer's disease. *Brain and Language* 28: 235–249.

Huff, F. Jacob, Mack, L., Mahlmann, J., and Greenberg, S. 1988. A comparison of lexical-semantic impairments in left hemisphere stroke and Alzheimer's disease. *Brain and Language* 34: 262–278.

Hutchinson, J. M. and Jensen, M. 1980. A pragmatic evaluation of discourse communication in normal and senile elderly in a nursing home. In L. Obler and M. Albert (eds.), *Language and Communication in the Elderly*, 59–73. Lexington, MA: Lexington Books.

Hymes, V. 1974. The ethnography of linguistic intuitions at Warm Springs. Paper presented at NWAVE III, Georgetown University, October 25, 1974.

Illes, J. 1989. Neurolinguistic features of spontaneous language production dissociate three forms of neurodegenerative disease: Alzheimer's, Huntington's, and Parkinson's. *Brain and Language* 37: 628–42.

Irigaray, L. 1973. *Le langage des dements*. The Hague: Mouton.

Kaplan, E., Goodglass, H., and Weintraub, S. 1983. *Boston Naming Test*. Philadelphia: Lea & Febiger.

Katz, I. 1981. *Stigma: A Social Psychological Analysis*. Hillsdale, NJ: Erlbaum.

Katzman, R. 1985. Current frontiers in research on Alzheimer's disease. In V. L. Melnick and N. N. Dubler (eds.), *Alzheimer's Dementia: Dilemmas in Clinical Research*, 1–11. Clifton, NJ: Humana Press.

1991. The diagnosis and treatment of Alzheimer's disease: What have we learned? Paper presented at the 44th Annual Scientific Meeting of the Gerontological Society of America, November 22–26, 1991. San Francisco.

Kempler, D. 1984. Syntactic and Symbolic Abilities in Alzheimer's Disease. Unpublished Ph.D. dissertation. Los Angeles: UCLA.

Kitwood, T. 1988. The technical, the personal, and the framing of dementia. *Social Behaviour* 3: 161–179.

Labov, W. 1972a. Some principles of linguistic methodology. *Language in Society* 1: 97–120.

1972b. The transformation of experience in narrative syntax. In W. Labov, *Sociolinguistic Patterns*. Philadelphia: University of Pennsylvania Press.

1972c. *Sociolinguistic Patterns*. Philadelphia: University of Pennsylvania Press.

1972d. The study of language in its social context. In P. Giglioli, *Language and Social Context*, 283–307. New York: Penguin Books.

Labov, W. and Fanshel, D. 1977. *Therapeutic Discourse*. New York: Academic Press.

Lakoff, R. 1973. The logic of politeness. *Chicago Linguistics Society*, 9: 292–305.

1979. Stylistic strategies within a grammar of style. In J. Orasanu, M. Slater, and L. L. Adler (eds.), *Language, Sex, and Gender*, 53–78. Annals of the New York Academy of Science 327.

Lehman, H. 1980. Schizophrenia. In H. Kaplan, A. Freedman, and B. Saddock (eds.), *Comprehensive Textbook of Psychiatry* III, 1104–1113, 1153–1192. Baltimore: Williams and Wilkins.

Lubinski, R. B. 1981. Language and aging: an environmental approach to intervention. *Topics in Language Disorders* 1: 89–97.

McCloskey, M. and Caramazza, A. 1988. Theory and methodology in cognitive neuropsychology: a response to our critics. *Cognitive Neuropsychology* 5: 583–623.

McDermott, R. P. and Tylbor, H. 1983. On the necessity of collusion in conversation. *Text* 3 (3): 277–297.

Mace, N. L. and Rabins, P. V. 1981. *The 36-Hour Day*. Baltimore: The Johns Hopkins University Press.

McTear, M. 1985. *Children's Conversation*. Oxford: Blackwell.

McTear, M. and King, F. 1991. Miscommunication in clinical contexts: the speech therapy interview. In N. Coupland, H. Giles, and J. Wiemann (eds.), *"Miscommunication" and Problematic Talk*, 195–214. Newbury Park: Sage Publications.

Martin, A. and Fedio, P. 1983. Word production and comprehension in Alzheimer's disease: the breakdown of semantic knowledge. *Brain and Language* 19: 124–141.

Mead, G. H. 1934. *Mind, Self, and Society*. University of Chicago Press.

Menn, L. and Obler, L. 1982. Exceptional language data as linguistic evidence: an introduction. In L. Obler and L. Menn (eds).), *Exceptional Language and Linguistics*, 3–14. New York: Academic Press.

Merritt, M. 1976. On questions following questions in service encounters. *Language in Society* 5: 315–357.

Miller, D. L. 1973. *George Herbert Mead: Self, Language and the World*. The University of Chicago Press.

Moeschler, J. 1986. Review article: answers to questions about questions and answers. *Journal of Pragmatics* 10: 227–253.

Moody, H. 1989. Gerontology with a human face. In L. E. Thomas (ed.), *Research on Adulthood and Aging*, 227–240. Albany: SUNY Press.

Murdoch, B. E., Chenery, H., Wilks, V., and Boyle, R. 1987. Language disorders in dementia of the Alzheimer type. *Brain and Language* 31: 122–137.

Murphy, G. L. 1990. The psycholinguistics of discourse comprehension. In Y. Joanette and H. H. Brownell (eds.), *Discourse Ability and Brain Damage*, 28–49. New York: Springer Verlag.

National Center for Health Statistics. 1985. *National Nursing Home Survey*. US Department of Health and Human Services.

Nebes, R. D. 1985. Preservation of semantic structure in dementia. In H. Ulatowska (ed.), *The Aging Brain*, 109–122. San Diego, CA: College-Hill Press.

Nebes, R. D., Martin, D. and Horn, L. 1984. Sparing of semantic memory in Alzheimer's disease. *Journal of Abnormal Psychology* 93 (3): 321–330.

Nicholas, M., Obler, L., Albert, M., and Helm-Estabrooks, N. 1985. Empty speech in Alzheimer's disease and fluent aphasia. *Journal of Speech and Hearing Research* 28: 405–410.

Nussbaum, J. F. 1991. Communication, language and the institutionalized elderly. *Ageing and Society* 11: 149–165.

Obler, L. 1981. Review of *Le langage des dements* by Luce Irigaray. *Brain and Language* 12: 375–386.

1983. Language and brain dysfunction in dementia. In S. Segalowitz (ed.), *Language Functions and Brain Organization*, 267–282. New York: Academic Press.

Obler, L. and Albert, M. 1980a. Language and aging: a neurobehavioral analysis. In D. S. Beasley and G. A. Davis (eds.), *Aging, Communication Processes and Disorders*, 107–121. New York: Grune and Stratton.

(eds.), 1980b. *Language and Communication in the Elderly: Clinical, Therapeutic, and Experimental Aspects*. Lexington, MA: Heath.

1981. Language in the elderly aphasic and in the dementing patient. In M. T. Sarno (ed.), *Acquired Aphasia*, 385–398. New York: Academic Press.

1984. Language in aging. In M. Albert (ed.), *Clinical Neurology of Aging*, 245–253. New York: Oxford.

Opit, L. J. 1988. The problem of senile dementia. *Social Behaviour* 3: 181–196.

Overman, C. and Goeffrey, V. 1987. Alzheimer's disease and other dementias. In H. G. Mueller and V. Goeffrey (eds.), *Communication Disorders in Aging*, 271–297. Washington, DC: Gallaudet University Press.

Parsons, T. 1951. *The Social System*. New York: The Free Press.

Pincus, L. 1981. *The Challenge of a Long Life*. London: Faber and Faber.

Price-Williams, D. and Sabsay, S. 1979. Communicative competence among severely retarded persons. *Semiotica* 26: 35–63.

Quirk, R., Greenbaum, S., Leech, G., and Svartvik, J. 1972. *A Grammar of Contemporary English*. London: Longman.

Reisberg, B. 1981. *A Guide to Alzheimer's Disease*. New York: The Free Press.

Reisberg, B., Ferris, S. H., de Leon, M. J. *et al.* 1982. The global deterioration scale (GDS): an instrument for the assessment of primary degenerative dementia (PDD). *American Journal of Psychiatry* 139: 1136–1139.

Richardson, A. P. and Marquandt, T. P. 1985. Language skills and communication breakdown in senile dementia. *Australian Journal of Human Communication Disorders* 13: 75–93.

Ripich, D. and Terrell, B. 1988. Patterns of discourse cohesion and coherence in Alzheimer's disease. *Journal of Speech and Hearing Disorders* 53: 8–15.

Ripich, D., Vertes, D., Whitehouse, P., Fulton, S., and Ekelman, B. 1991. Turn-taking and speech act patterns in the discourse of senile dementia of the Alzheimer's type patients. *Brain and Language* 40: 330–343.

Robinson, W. P. and S. J. Rackstraw. 1972. *A Question of Answers*. 2 vols. London.

Rosen, H. 1988. The autobiographical impulse. In D. Tannen (ed.), *Linguistics in Context*. Norwood, NJ: Ablex.

Rust, L. 1986. Another part of the country. In J. Alexander, D. Berrow, L. Domitrovich, M. Donnelly, and C. McLean (eds.), *Women and Aging*. Corvallis, Oregon: Calyx Books.

Sabat, S. 1991. Turn-taking, turn-giving, and Alzheimer's disease. *Georgetown Journal of Languages and Linguistics* 2: 161–175.

Sabat, S., Wiggs, C., and Pinizzotto, A. 1984. Alzheimer's disease: clinical vs. observational studies of cognitive ability. *Journal of Clinical Experimental Gerontology* 6: 337–359.

Sabsay, S. and Platt, M. 1985. Weaving the cloak of competence: a paradox in the management of trouble in conversations between retarded and nonretarded interlocutors. In S. Sabsay, M. Platt, *et al.* (eds.), *Social Setting, Stigma and Communicative Competence*, 95–119. Amsterdam: John Benjamins.

Sacks, H., Schegloff, E., and Jefferson, G. 1978. A simplest systematics for the orgnaization of turn-taking for conversation. In J. Schenkein (ed.), *Studies in the Organization of Conversational Interaction*, 7–55. New York: Academic Press. (Paper first published in *Language* 50 [1974].)

Sacks, O. 1987. *The Man who Mistook His Wife for a Hat and Other Clinical Tales*. New York: Harper and Row, Publishers.

St. Claire, L. 1986. Mental retardation: impairment or handicap? *Disability, Handicap & Society* 1: 233–243.

    1989. A multi-dimensional model of mental retardation: impairment, subnormal behaviour, role failures and socially constructed retardation. *American Journal of Mental Retardation* 94: 88–96.

Sandson, J., Obler, L., and Albert, M. 1987. Language changes in healthy aging and dementia. In Rosenberg, Sheldon (ed.), *Advances in Applied Psycholinguistics*, vol. I. Cambridge University Press.

Schegloff, E. 1968. Sequencing in conversational openings. *American Anthropologist* 70: 1075–1095.

    1978. On some questions and ambiguities in conversation. In W. Dressler (ed.), *Current Trends in Text Linguistics*, 81–102. Berlin: de Gruyter.

Schegloff, E. and Sacks, H. 1973. Opening up closings. *Semiotica* 8: 289–327.

Schegloff, E., Jefferson, G., and Sacks, H. 1977. The preference for self-correction in the organization of repair in conversation. *Language* 53, 361–82.

Schiffrin, D. 1985. Conversational coherence: the role of *well*. *Language* 61: 640–667.

    1987. *Discourse Markers*. Cambridge University Press.

    1991. Conversation analysis. *Annual Review of Applied Linguistics (1990)* 11: 3–16.

Scott, M. and Lyman, S. 1968. Accounts. *American Sociological Review*, 46–62.

Schwartz, M. F., Marin, O., and Saffran, E. 1979. Dissociations of language function in dementia: a case study. *Brain and Language* 7: 277–306.

Searle, J. 1969. *Speech Acts*. Cambridge University Press.

    1975. Indirect speech acts. In P. Cole and J. Morgan (eds.), *Speech Acts*, Syntax and Semantics vol. III, 59–82. New York: Academic Press.

Shekim, L. O. 1983. Production of Discourse in Individuals with Alzheimer's Disease. Unpublished Ph.D. Dissertation. University of Florida.

Shindler. A. G., Caplan, L. R., and Hier, D. B. 1984. Intrusions and perseverations. *Brain and Language* 23: 148–158.

Shuttleworth, E. and Huber, S. 1988. The naming disorder of dementia of Alzheimer type. *Brain and Language* 34: 222–234.

Simmel, G. 1961 [1911]. The sociology of sociability. In T. Parsons *et al.* (eds.), *Theories of Society*, 157–162. New York: The Free Press.

Sloan, P. 1990a. The normal brain: an overview. In R. Hamdy, J. Turnbull, L. Norman, and M. Lancaster (eds.), *Alzheimer's Disease: A Handbook for Caregivers*, 208–220. St. Louis: The C.V. Mosby Company.

    1990b. Neuropsychological assessment of dementia. In R. Hamdy, J. Turnbull,

L. Norman, and M. Lancaster (eds.), *Alzheimer's Disease: A Handbook for Caregivers*, 221–240. St. Louis: The C.V. Mosby Company.

Smith, C. and Ventis, D. 1990. Cooperative and supportive conversational behavior of female Alzheimer's patients. Paper presented at the 43rd Annual Scientific Meeting of the Gerontological Society of America, November 17. Boston, MA.

Smith, S. R., Chenery, H., and Murdoch, B. 1989. Semantic abilities in dementia of the Alzheimer type II: Grammatical semantics. *Brain and Language* 36: 533–542.

Smithers, J. 1977. Dimensions of senility. *Urban Life* 6: 251–276.

Stenström, A.-B. 1984. *Questions and Responses in English Conversation*. Malmö: Cwk Gleerup.

Stevens, S. 1985. The language of dementia in the elderly: a pilot study. *British Journal of Disorders of Communication* 20: 181–190.

Storandt, M. 1987. Relationship of normal aging and dementing diseases of aged. Group Report 4 of the Dahlem Workshop on the Etiology of Dementia of Alzheimer Type, December 7–11, Berlin.

Stubbs, M. 1983. *Discourse Analysis*. University of Chicago Press.

Tannen, D. 1981. Review of *Therapeutic Discourse* by William Labov and David Fanshel (1977). *Language* 57: 481–496.

1984. *Conversational Style*. Norwood, NJ: Ablex.

1987a. Repetition in conversation as spontaneous formulaicity. *Text* 7: 215–243.

1987b. Repetition in conversation: towards a poetics of talk. *Language* 63: 574–604.

1989. *Talking Voices: Repetition, Dialogue, and Imagery in Conversational Discourse*. Cambridge University Press.

Terry, R. 1991. The post-mortem examination: insights into the origin of Alzheimer's disease. Paper presented at the 44th Annual Scientific Meeting of the Gerontological Society of America, November 22–26. San Francisco.

Terry, R. and Katzman, R. 1983. Senile dementia of the Alzheimer type. *Annals of Neurology* 14: 497–506.

Tulving, E. 1972. Episodic and semantic memory. In E. Tulving and W. Donaldson (eds.), *Organization of Memory*, 381–403. New York: Academic Press.

Tyack, D. and Ingram, D. 1977. Children's production and comprehension of questions. *Journal of Child Language* 4: 211–224.

Ulatowska, H., Allard, L., Donnell, A., Bristow, J., Hayes, S., Flower, A., and North, A. 1988. Discourse performance in subjects with dementia of the Alzheimer type. In H. Whitaker (ed.), *Neuropsychological Studies of Nonfocal Brain Damage*, 108–131. New York: Springer Verlag.

Ulatowska H., Allard, L. and Chapman, S. 1990. Narrative and procedural discourse in aphasia. In Y. Joannette and H. Brownell (eds.), *Discourse Ability and Brain Damage*, 180–198. New York: Springer Verlag.

US Office of Technology Assessment. 1992. *Special Care Units for People with Alzheimer's and Other Dementias*.

Weinreich, U., Labov, W., and Herzog, M. 1968. Empirical foundations for a theory of language change. In W. Lehmann and Y. Malkiel (eds.), *Directions for Historical Linguistics*. Austin: University of Texas Press.

Wertz, R. 1978. Neuropathologies of speech and language: an introduction to patient management. In D. F. Johns (ed.), *Clinical Management of Neurogenetic Communicative Disorders*, 1–101. Boston: Little, Brown and Company.

Whitaker. H. 1982a. Automatization of language. Lecture given at Georgetown University, March.

1982b. Automaticity. Paper presented at the Conference on Formulaicity, Linguistic Institute, University of Maryland.

Wiemann, J. M., Gravell, R., and Wiemann, M. C. 1990. Communication with the elderly: implications for health care and social support. In H. Giles, N. Coupland, and J. M. Wiemann (eds.), *Communication, Health and the Elderly*, 1–28. Manchester University Press.

Williams, A. and Giles, H. 1991. Sociopsychological perspectives on older people's language and communication. *Ageing and Society* 11: 103–126.

Wood, P. H. N. and Badley, E. M. 1978a. Setting disablement in perspective. *International Rehabilitation Medicine*, 1: 32–37.

1978b. An epidemiological appraisal of disablement. In A. E. Bennett (ed.), *Recent Advances in Community Medicine*. Edinburgh: Churchill Livingstone.

1980. *People with Disabilities*. World Rehabilitation Fund, Inc.

Wood, L. and Ryan, E. 1991. Talk to elders: social structure, attitudes and forms of address. *Ageing and Society* 11: 167–187.

Yadugiri, M. A. 1986. Some pragmatic implications of the use of *yes* and *no* in response to *yes–no* questions. *Journal of Pragmatics* 10: 199–210.

Index

183